POCKET GUIDE TO
Pediatric
Fractures

POCKET GUIDE TO
Pediatric
Fractures

JOHN A. OGDEN, M.D.

Chief of Staff
Shriners Hospitals for Crippled Children
Tampa, Florida

Professor of Orthopaedics
Department of Orthopaedic Surgery
University of South Florida, College of Medicine
Tampa, Florida

Clinical Professor of Orthopaedics
Yale University School of Medicine
New Haven, Connecticut

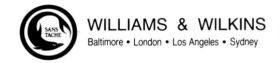

WILLIAMS & WILKINS
Baltimore • London • Los Angeles • Sydney

Editor: Kimberly Kist
Associate Editor: Linda Napora
Copy Editor: Brenda Brienza
Design: JoAnne Janowiak
Illustration Planning: Wayne Hubbel
Production: Raymond E. Reter

Printed in the United States of America

Library of Congress Cataloging-in-Publication Data

Main entry under title:

Ogden, John A. (John Anthony), 1942–
  Pocket guide to pediatric fractures.

  Includes bibliographies and index.
  1. Fractures in children—Handbooks, manuals, etc. 2. Dislocations in children—Handbooks, manuals, etc. I. Title. [DNLM: 1. Dislocations—in infancy & childhood—handbooks. 2. Fractures—in infancy & childhood—handbooks. WE 39 034p]
  RD101.034 1987   617'.16   86-30769
  ISBN 0-683-06637-4

87 88 89 90 91
10 9 8 7 6 5 4 3 2 1

To my parents

To Dali

To Stephanie and John III

Preface

Injury from birth through adolescence is a part of the trials and tribulations of growing, exploring, and enjoying one's enlarging environment. Yet the extent of injury possible and the highly variable, often unique injuries of the developing skeleton frequently make diagnosis and treatment difficult.

The goal of this book is to provide a basic guide for the medical student and house officer, whether he or she is going to be a family practitioner, pediatrician, radiologist, general surgeon, or orthopaedist. This book should enable each to recognize the basics of diagnosis, to be able to render excellent *initial* care, and to be aware of potential short-term and long-term complications. This book is not meant to be detailed. Rather, the reader should be directed to more definitive works by the author and others, such as, J Ogden, *Skeletal Injury in the Child* (Lea and Febiger, Philadelphia) and C Rockwood, K Wilkins, R King, (eds.), *Fractures; Children*, Vol. 3 (JB Lippincott, Philadelphia).

I hope this book will serve as an introduction for those most often involved in the initial evaluation of the injured child, and that this will, accordingly, help further the better diagnosis and subsequent treatment of fractures in children of all ages.

I would like to extend my sincere appreciation to Richard Remington for the pen and ink drawings; Patricia Glas Cosgrove, Janet Barber, and Wendie Smith for the photography; and Marguerite Treep and Shirley Gauthier for the innumerable drafts necessary to create this book. I would also like to thank the Board of Governors of the Tampa Unit and the National Trustees of the Shriners Hospitals for Crippled Children, especially Robert J. Turley and Gene Bracewell for the support they have given in their constant efforts to bring excellent care to children with orthopaedic and burn injuries and diseases.

Sachem's Head
Branford College   John A. Ogden, M.D.

Contents

Preface vii
General Principles 1
Radiologic Aspects 14
Growth Mechanism Injury—General Aspects 22
Growth Mechanism Injury—Type 1 24
Growth Mechanism Injury—Type 2 26
Growth Mechanism Injury—Type 3 30
Growth Mechanism Injury—Type 4 32
Growth Mechanism Injury—Type 5 34
Growth Mechanism Injury—Type 6 36
Growth Mechanism Injury—Type 7 38
Growth Mechanism Injury—Type 8 40
Growth Mechanism Injury—Type 9 42
Neonatal Fractures 44
Myelodysplasia 46
Osteogenesis Imperfecta 48
Head Injury 49
Stress Fractures 50
Child Abuse 52
Clavicle—Proximal 54
Clavicle—Diaphysis 56
Clavicle—Distal 58

Shoulder—Dislocation 60
Humerus—Proximal Epiphysis 62
Humerus—Proximal Metaphysis 64
Humerus—Diaphysis 66
Humerus—Supracondylar (Distal Metaphysis) 68
Humerus—Transcondylar (Physeal) 72
Humerus—Lateral Condyle 74
Humerus—Medial Condyle 78
Humerus—Lateral Epicondyle 80
Humerus—Medial Epicondyle 82
Elbow—"Little League Elbow" 84
Elbow—Dislocation 86
Elbow—"Nursemaid's Elbow" 90
Proximal Ulna 92
Proximal Radius 94
Monteggia Injury 96
Radius and Ulna—Diaphysis (Bowing) 98
Radius and Ulna—Diaphysis (Greenstick) 100
Radius and Ulna—Diaphysis (One Bone) 102
Radius and Ulna—Diaphysis (Both Bones) 104
Radius and Ulna—Distal Metaphysis 106
Radius—Distal Physis 108
Ulna—Distal Physis 110
Wrist—Carpal Navicular 112
Thumb—Dislocation 114
Thumb—Bennett's Fracture 116
Hand—Metacarpal Fracture (Diaphysis) 118
Hand—Metacarpal Fracture (Distal) 120
Hand—Metacarpophalangeal Dislocation 122
Hand—Phalangeal Physis 124
Hand—Extra-Octave Fracture 128
Hand—Interphalangeal Dislocation 130

Hand—Phalanx (Condyle) 132
Hand—Mallet Finger 134
Hand—Distal Phalanx (Tuft) 136
Spine—C1 138
Spine—C1/C2 Rotational Subluxation 140
Spine—C2 142
Spine—Lower Cervical 144
Spine—Thoracolumbar 148
Spine—Lumbar Apophysis 150
Pelvis—Rami 152
Pelvis—Acetabulum (Triradiate Cartilage) 154
Pelvis—Iliac Spines 156
Pelvis—Ischium 158
Hip—Dislocation 160
Femur—Proximal Physis 162
Femur—Slipped Capital Femoral Epiphysis 164
Femur—Femoral Neck 166
Femur—Greater Trochanter 168
Femur—Lesser Trochanter 170
Femur—Subtrochanteric Fracture 172
Femur—Diaphysis 174
Femur—Distal Metaphysis 176
Femur—Distal Physis 178
Knee—Osteochondral Injury 182
Knee—Dislocation 184
Knee—Patellar Dislocation 186
Knee—Patellar Subluxation 188
Knee—Collateral Ligaments 190
Knee—Patellar Fracture 192
Knee—Distal Patella 194
Knee—Meniscal Injury 196
Tibia/Fibula—Tibial Spines 198

Tibia/Fibula—Proximal Epiphysis 200

Tibia/Fibula—Tibial Tuberosity 202

Tibia/Fibula—Osgood-Schlatter's Lesion 204

Tibia/Fibula—Proximal Fibula 206

Tibia/Fibula—Proximal Fibular Dislocation 208

Tibia/Fibula—Proximal Metaphysis 210

Tibia/Fibula—Diaphysis 212

Tibia/Fibula—Toddler's Fracture 214

Tibia/Fibula—Distal Metaphysis 216

Tibia/Fibula—Distal Epiphysis (Types 1 and 2) 218

Tibia/Fibula—Distal Epiphysis (Triplane) 220

Tibia/Fibula—Distal Epiphysis (Tillaux) 222

Tibia/Fibula—Distal Epiphysis (Malleoli) 224

Foot—Puncture Wounds 226

Foot—Talus 228

Foot—Calcaneus 230

Foot—Tarsal Coalition 232

Foot—Navicula 234

Foot—Metatarsals 236

Foot—Proximal Fifth Metatarsal 238

Foot—Phalanges 240

Index 243

General Principles

Skeletal injuries account for 10 to 15% of all childhood injuries. Any physician treating childhood skeletal injuries should be familiar with the probable mechanism of injury, the short-term and long-term biologic responses of the injured part, especially when a growth mechanism is involved, and the appropriate guidelines for treatment of the specific injury. Since these skeletally immature patients have all of their productive years ahead of them, they must be treated with skills based upon a detailed knowledge of the capacities of repair and remodeling. If a physician relies only upon principles of treatment applicable to injuries of the adult skeleton, errors in judgment and technique may manifest in permanent defects.

The differences between the injured bones of an adult and a child relate to the child's skeletal components being in a more dynamic, constantly changing growth mode, whereas the adult skeleton has ceased elongation and apposition, and is principally remodeling the established elements in accord with biologic stress responses.

Because of progressive endochondral ossification, the chondroosseous epiphyses of children are variably radiolucent, making evaluation difficult, if not impossible, unless specific procedures such as arthrography are used. Skeletal injury sometimes must be inferred on the basis of clinical judgment, for roentgenographic substantiation may not be immediately possible. However, subsequent new bone formation may make the diagnosis certain.

The physes are constantly changing their contributions to longitudinal and diametric growth and their mechanical relations to other components. Patterns of failure thus vary with the degree of chondroosseous maturation. The child's periosteum is thicker, more readily elevated from the diaphyseal and metaphyseal bone, less readily com-

1

pletely disrupted, and exhibits greater osteogenic potential than the same tissue following skeletal maturation. Developing bone begins with fewer lamellar components and a relatively greater porosity than mature bone. Within any given anatomic region of a bone, changes gradually occur. The natural sequence begins with increased lamellar bone being formed in the diaphysis. There are also relative differences in the various regions within a given bone that predispose certain regions to fracture over others. These differences in microscopic and macroscopic architecture also affect the process of fracture healing, which is different in the more dense, lamellar bone of the diaphysis, as compared to the spongy, trabecular bone of the metaphysis or epiphysis.

The skeleton is undergoing active, frequently rapid, growth and remodeling. Accordingly, fractures usually heal rapidly, non-union is rare, overgrowth is common, and certain angular deformities may correct totally. However, damage to the capacity of the bone to accomplish normal physiologic functions may impair subsequent growth and development in several ways. Various portions of the longitudinal bones respond differently to hormones, mechanical factors, vascular changes, and trauma.

The major change in developing bone is increasing density of the cortical bone in the diaphysis and metaphysis. The cross-sectional porosity of a child's bone is much greater than that of an adult and may limit fracture propagation. This factor undoubtedly is important, since comminuted fractures are uncommon in children. The increased amount of bone in the epiphyseal ossification center undoubtedly alters the stress/strain response pattern of the epiphysis, and it is likely that establishment of the subchondral plate over the physis alters its response to fracture. Adult bone usually fails in tension, whereas a child's bone may fail in either tension or compression.

Satisfactory diagnosis and initial treatment necessitate an understanding of what comprises each specific fracture. A fracture is the disruption of the normal continuity of the bone and/or cartilage. The disruption may or may not cause a break in the continuity of the cortical bone, a factor that can occur in children when the developing cortical bone, because of a greater capacity for plastic deformation prior to failure, buckles rather than breaks. This represents compression failure, rather than tensile failure of bone, and can occur only in children. Tensile failure, which certainly may occur in children and is the prevailing mode of failure in adults, usually leads to a break in structural continuity of the bone.

Each fracture needs to be described adequately. Such a description should include: (1) the anatomic location of the fracture; (2) the type of fracture; and (3) the physical changes caused by and associated with the fracture. Proper description obviously allows better communication between the primary care and the consulting physicians.

ANATOMIC LOCATION

Terminology locates the injury accurately. Slight differences in anatomic locale of the fracture in children may have a major impact on acute treatment and potential long-term problems. These definitions are illustrated in Figure 1:

Diaphyseal

Involvement of the central shaft of a longitudinal bone, which is progressively composed of mature, lamellar bone.

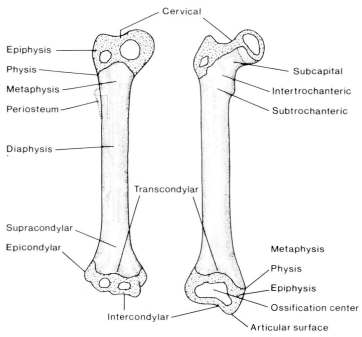

Figure 1. Anatomic references usually used to localize fractures involving developing bone.

Metaphyseal

Involvement of the flaring ends of the central shaft of a longitudinal bone. The metaphyses are usually composed of extensive endosteal trabecular bone and cortical immature fiber bone, both of which predispose the metaphyses to the torus fracture.

Physeal

Involvement of the endochondral growth mechanism.

Epiphyseal

Involvement of the chondro-osseous end of a long bone. It is important to realize that the epiphysis may be injured *only* in the cartilaginous portion, which may make diagnosis extremely difficult.

Articular

Involvement of the epiphyseal region that has formed the joint surface. The injury may be part of a more extensive epiphyseal injury, or it may be localized. In the latter case, the fragment may include only articular cartilage and juxtaposed, undifferentiated hyaline cartilage, or both subchondral bone and cartilage.

Epicondylar

Involvement of regions of the bone, especially around the elbow, that serve as major muscle attachments and have extensions of the physis and epiphysis.

Subcapital

Involvement just below the epiphyses of certain bones such as the proximal femur or radius.

Cervical

Involvement along the neck of a specific bone, such as the proximal humerus or femur.

Supracondylar

Involvement above the level of the condyles and epicondyles (e.g., distal humerus).

Transcondylar

Located transversely across the condyles, this usually is a physeal fracture of the distal humerus or femur.

Intercondylar

Involvement of the epiphysis, with fracture separating the normal condylar anatomic relationships.

Malleolar

Involvement of the distal regions of the fibula and tibia. Because of anatomic differences, there are significant differences in the fracture patterns of the medial and lateral malleoli.

TYPES OF FRACTURES

The basic fracture patterns, shown in Figure 2, are as follows:

Longitudinal

The fracture line follows the longitudinal axis of the diaphysis.

Transverse

The fracture line is at a right angle to the longitudinal axis.

Oblique

The fracture line is variably angled relative to the longitudinal axis, usually about 30 to 45 degrees.

Spiral

The fracture line is oblique and encircles a portion of the shaft.

Impacted

This is a compression type injury in which the cortical and trabecular bone of each side of the fracture are crushed.

Comminuted

The fracture line propagates in several directions, creating multiple, variable-sized fragments.

Bowing

The bone is deformed beyond its capacity for full elastic recoil into permanent plastic deformation. The younger the child, the more likely it is that this type of skeletal injury will occur. It is common in the fibula and the ulna, both of which may bow while the paired bone (i.e., tibia or radius) fractures. This permanent deformation may limit the reducibility of the fractured bone of the pair.

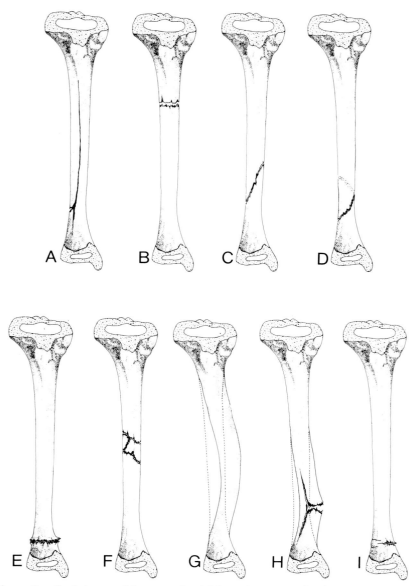

Figure 2. Basic types of fractures in children. A. Longitudinal B. Transverse. C. Oblique. D. Spiral. E. Impacted. F. Comminuted. G. Bowing. H. Greenstick. I. Torus.

Greenstick

This is a common injury in children. The bone is completely fractured, with a portion of the cortex and periosteum remaining intact on the compression side. Since this intact cortical bone is usually plastically deformed (bowed), an angular deformity is common, which may necessitate conversion to a complete fracture by reversal of the deformity.

Torus

This is an impaction injury. Because of the differing response of the metaphyseal bone to a compression load, the bone buckles, rather than fracturing completely, and a relatively stable injury is created.

PHYSICAL CHANGE

While the aforementioned terms have been primarily descriptive, the following terms describe conditions that are of practical importance. These terms indicate not only the nature of the clinical problem, but also the general type of treatment that will be required.

Extent

The fracture may be incomplete, in which case some of the cortex is intact, or it may be complete, in which case the fracture line crosses the entire circumference. Further, the fracture line may be simple (a single fracture line), segmental (separate fracture lines isolating a segment of bone), or comminuted (multiple fracture lines and fragments).

Relationship of Fracture Fragments to Each Other (Fig. 3)

These relationships define a deformity as it exists during the roentgenographic evaluation. However, because of elastic recoil in children, these relationships may not represent the full extent of deformity present at the time of injury. The fracture may appear undisplaced or displaced, in which case the distal fragment is shifted away from its usual relationship to the proximal fragment. This shift may assume several types of deformation, which may be present singly or in any combination. These are: (1) sideways shift, (2) angulation, (3) overriding, (4) distraction, (5) shortening, and (6) rotation. The most important changes to correct are angular and rotational deformities. As long as the reduction emphasizes restoration of longitudinal and rotational alignment, sideways shifts and overriding may be acceptable. Rotational deformities *must* be corrected.

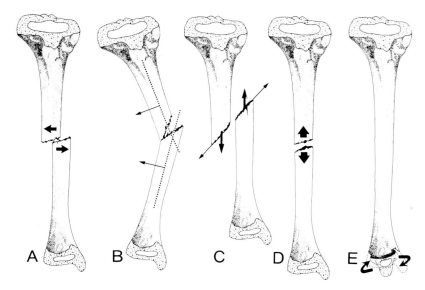

Figure 3. Relationships of fracture fragments to each other. A. Lateral displacement. B. Angular displacement. C. Overriding. D. Distraction. E. Rotational displacement.

Relationship of Fracture to External Environment

Basically, a fracture is either closed (skin intact) or open (compound). An open fracture which allows a communication between the fracture and the external environment, may be caused by a fracture fragment penetrating the skin from within or by an external object penetrating the skin. Such fractures have a serious risk of infection to the bone and contiguous soft tissues.

BASICS OF TREATMENT

Children require different and often specialized treatment. They have smaller respiratory and circulatory volumes, different responses to drugs, surgery, and stress, and frequent difficulty in localizing and communicating symptoms. The response of the injured child is different physiologically and psychologically from an adult. The loss of a small amount of blood is proportionately more significant because of the child's lessened overall blood volume. The relatively large surface area, compared to body weight, allows rapid heat and water losses.

The problems requiring immediate attention in the management of a severely injured child are not different from those of the adult. Establishment and maintenance of an adequate airway, control of hemorrhage, detection and evaluation of head injury, replacement of blood loss, treatment of shock, recognition of serious skeletal injuries, and the prevention of further injury through judicious and expeditious handling are of prime importance.

Before satisfactory treatment can be provided, the apprehensions of the child must be dispelled, and appropriate pain relief given. If reduction is necessary, proper levels of sedation and/or anesthesia are essential. Local anesthetic infiltration of the fracture site may increase the risk of infection. Intravenous regional block or even selective nerve blocks may be accomplished in older children. The use of intravenous agents (e.g., diazepam) must be undertaken with caution. Appropriate anesthetic equipment must be available (mask, oxygen source, etc.). Further, one must remember that diazepam is basically an amnesic, not an analgesic agent. The child will feel and react to pain, but will not remember doing so. The drug response may be delayed. Any child being sent to another area for post reduction films must be appropriately alert or respiratory arrest may occur in an area where observation and resuscitation are difficult.

In any fracture requiring muscle relaxation for reduction, a general anesthetic is more useful. This is particularly true for supracondylar humeral and dorsally displaced distal radial fractures. If general anesthesia is used, the child often should be admitted to the hospital for overnight observation of not only recovery from anesthesia but also of the peripheral neurovascular response to the injury, since displacement and manipulative reduction, which may be difficult, are certainly a further trauma to the already injured tissues.

The basic principle of fracture reduction is reversal of the mechanism of injury. Reduction by this method, however, depends on the presence of the soft-tissue linkage (Fig. 4). Another step in fracture treatment is to align the fragment you can control more easily. Usually the distal fragment can be controlled more easily, and it should be aligned longitudinally with the proximal fragment. The proximal fragment adopts a position dictated by the pull of the muscles attached to it.

Closed reduction is adequate to maintain normal alignment of most fractures in children, because the plastic remodeling of their bones engenders good final anatomic and functional results. Rotational deformities must be corrected. Except in those fractures involving joints and epiphyses, absolute anatomic reduction of the bone fragments is

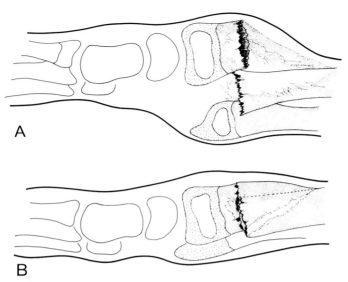

Figure 4. These schematic drawings depict a typical dorsally displaced distal radial fracture. The relatively thick, osteogenic periosteum usually is partially intact (A) and may be used to provide an intrinsic stability during reduction, with callus rapidly forming between it and the metaphysis (B).

not always necessary, and sometimes should be purposely avoided. Angulation in the middle third of long bones is unacceptable, and should be corrected as close to normal as possible. Direct apposition of bone ends is less important. Bayonet (side-to-side) apposition, especially in the midfemur, is desirable and leads to prompt, strong osseous union. After injury, the bones of children may grow at an accelerated rate for six to eight months. Overgrowth is a complication of some childhood fractures that may be avoided if general principles of treatment are understood. The younger the child, the greater the amount of anticipated remodeling.

Some physicians emphatically condemn internal fixation of fractures in childhood, suggesting that non-union, delayed union, altered growth, infection, and ugly scars may arise. While it is certainly correct that the thoughtless use of internal fixation should be strongly discouraged in treating fractures in children, it is incorrect to deny such application altogether. A useful guide is that operative treatment should be used when closed reduction cannot achieve an acceptable result. Open reduction and internal fixation are commonly indicated as an appropriate methodology in fracture separations of the capitellum, trochlea, and the medial epicondylar regions. Because of histologic differences between the bone of children and adults, rigid compression fixation is not always necessary. Fixation devices may be considered as methods of maintaining anatomic alignment in a bone that will heal rapidly with or without direct compression.

Fractures of the shaft of the radius and ulna usually may be managed conservatively, but when there are exceptions, such as severely damaged bone and soft tissue, that may result in complete loss of intrinsic stability, open reduction should be considered, particularly for older children. Complete fractures of the shaft of the ulna with dislocation of the radial head provide an important indication for surgery. Fractures of the neck of the femur are best treated by fixation with multiple pins.

At any age, complicating factors such as burns, spasticity (developmental or due to head injury), or multiple osseous injuries, have an effect on treatment. For instance, fractures of the femoral shaft may be treated more satisfactorily by internal fixation in cases involving hypertonicity due to head trauma. The potential calamities of non-union and infection should be avoidable through good surgical technique with prophylactic antibiotic treatment. Growth abnormalities should not occur if the vulnerability of the epiphyseal growth plates, both peripherally and centrally, is respected. Fixation plates should always be removed after satisfactory healing has occurred. External fixation devices also may be applied effectively in children, as long as the growth regions are not violated by the pins.

Many types of fractures of the physis and epiphysis are best treated by immediate open reduction and internal fixation. However, open reduction may be dangerous if performed several days or weeks after the epiphyseal injury because the danger of damage to the growth plate increases. If displacement is still severe and open reduction is necessary, the surgeon can lessen, if not altogether avoid, these risks by handling the region around the growth plate with extreme care.

Because children devise ingenious methods for destroying immobilization devices, casts or splints must be applied securely. As a general rule, one or more joints on either side of the fracture should be immobilized. Follow-up radiographs should be obtained at about five to ten days following reduction. During this time, the reactive swelling and pain are subsiding and the child's activity level is increasing, so the cast may loosen and cause the reduction to be lost. This is also the period during which a loss of reduction or a less acceptable angulation is easiest to correct.

Physical therapy in the otherwise normal child has a negligible role. Active use of the part by the child is almost always superior to the use of passive exercise by a therapist. Exaggerated limps gradually disappear and stiff elbows loosen, even if indifferent attention is paid to this phase of treatment. Normal use will invariably permit a return of motion. In the child, residual loss of motion probably is caused in part by anatomic malunion, and this will never be corrected by aggressive physical therapy. The therapist does play a major role, however, in rehabilitation of the child with a functional disability. In addition, children with neuromuscular disorders, such as cerebral palsy and myelomeningocele, sometimes require extensive physical therapy to attain pre-injury activity levels, since trauma may cause significant regression of limb function.

Children's fractures do not always remodel, and results are sometimes unacceptable. The remodeling capacity of a deformity caused by a fracture or epiphyseal injury is determined by three basic factors: (1) the age of the child; (2) the distance of the fracture from the end of the bone; and (3) the amount of angulation. The physiologic remodeling of a bone depends on periosteal appositional bone formation, resorption of some bone, and epiphyseal growth.

Remodeling is not something that can be totally or predictably relied upon, and every effort should be expended to attain as adequate an anatomic reduction as possible. Remodeling, in general, may be counted on in children with two or more years of growth after the injury, in children with fractures within the metaphyses, and in children with deformities in the plane of movement of the contiguous joint. In contrast, remodeling will not help with displaced intra-articular fractures, fractures toward the middle of the shaft of a bone (particularly when shortened, angulated, or rotated), displaced fractures where the axis of displacement is at a right angle to the normal plane of movement, and displaced fractures crossing the growth plate. Remodeling in the diaphysis is largely a process of smoothing the bone, as evident in follow-up radiographs; it is not necessarily a true correction of longitudinal alignment. In fractures of the shaft, the periosteum drapes one side of the bone and this gradually fills in, whereas the other side is bare or denuded of normal periosteum and resorbs to some degree. This makes the fracture look less obvious when, in reality, there is minimal improvement in the alignment. Near an epiphysis, however, the growth plate can realign and assume a more normal growth pattern by means of which metaphyseal remodeling will improve the overall appearance.

Potential complications differ in children and adults due to state of growth of the skeleton. Delayed union and non-union are rare in children, because the healing capacity is better. Post traumatic joint stiffness is uncommon if the joint itself is not directly damaged. Mechanical hindrance due to malunion of the fracture rarely exists, sometimes being present in supracondylar fractures of the humerus. Refractures and myositis ossificans are less common in children than in adults, and there is a specific problem of injury to the growth area.

References

Hanlon CR, Estes WL: Fractures in childhood—a statistical analysis. Am J Surg 87:312, 1954.

Ogden JA: Injury to the immature skeleton. In Touloukian RJ, (ed): Pediatric Trauma. New York, John Wiley & Sons, Inc., 1978.

Ogden JA: Skeletal Injury in the Child. Philadelphia, Lea and Febiger, 1982.

Ogden JA: The uniqueness of growing bones. In Rockwood CA Jr, Wilkins KE, King RE (eds): Fractures, Children (Vol 3). Philadelphia, JB Lippincott, 1984.

Ogden JA, Grogan DP, Light TR: The prenatal and postnatal development and growth of the musculoskeletal system. In Albright JA, Brand RA (eds): The Scientific Basis of Orthopaedics (2nd ed). New York, Appleton-Century-Crofts, 1987.

Rang M: Children's Fractures (2nd ed). Philadelphia, JB Lippincott, 1981.

Rockwood C, Wilkins K, King R (eds): Fractures, Children (Vol. 3). Philadelphia, JB Lippincott, 1983.

Ryoppy S: Injuries of the growing skeleton. Ann Chir Gynaecol Fenn 61:3, 1972.

Weber BG, Brunner C, Freuler F, eds: Treatment of Fractures in Children and Adolescents. Berlin, Springer-Verlag, 1980.

Radiologic Aspects

Radiology is essential for the evaluation of chondro-osseous trauma. However, fractures in children are not always easy to visualize radiographically. Roentgenograms must be of sufficiently good technical quality to elucidate not only the osseous injury, but also the normal and distorted soft tissue contours and the intra-articular fat-fluid levels (in appropriate cases). Technically poor films should never be accepted. Standard positional radiographs (anteroposterior and lateral) must be supplemented, as indicated, with appropriate oblique views and special procedures.

The roentgenographic evaluation of chondro-osseous injury must be based on a thorough knowledge of changing anatomy and response patterns in the developing skeleton. The importance of an orderly approach to the differential diagnosis of childhood skeletal trauma cannot be overemphasized. Even in the case of a simple fracture, care must be taken to thoroughly evaluate other areas, such as the joints on either side of the injury, the soft tissues, and the extent of the injury to the opposite of two paired bones when one is not obviously fractured. In particular, it is easy to overlook plastic deformation of the ulna or fibula, or dislocation of the radial or fibular head, any of which may cause significant difficulties in anatomic reduction, healing, and subsequent rehabilitation, and lead to growth deformity.

Usually a bone must be visualized in at least two views, these ideally being anteroposterior and lateral projections 90 degrees apart. Nonstandard projections, while sometimes unavoidable because of pain, displacement, or limitation of motion, may be misleading. Improperly positioned films may place the physis in an unusual projection, making it appear fractured to the inexperienced eye. It is imperative that the joints on either side of a fracture be radiographed so that the complete chondro-osseous unit(s) can be seen. Dislocations, especially those of the hip or radial head, are not uncommon in association with diaphyseal fractures.

The injured extremity must be adequately splinted and protected prior to sending the child for roentgenographic evaluation. The physician should state that the *entire* arm be rotated to assess a forearm fracture. Otherwise, the technician may simply turn the unprotected distal region 90 degrees, leaving the rest of the arm in the original position. This problem is particularly encountered in supracondylar humeral fractures.

Since the radiographic appearance of epiphyseal injuries may be subtle, the inexperienced observer may not recognize the injury. Sometimes a comparison view is necessary. Unfortunately, it has become routine practice in some hospitals and offices to obtain comparison views of the contralateral extremity as a way of differentiating fractures from developmental variations. This generally is unnecessary, particularly when the films are interpreted by someone with sufficient experience. In most cases, this practice only exposes the child to unnecessary additional radiation. Furthermore, there may be asymmetric epiphyseal ossification centers which might confuse, rather than clarify. When an inexperienced observer must make the immediate interpretation of the film, or when sufficient doubt exists, comparison films may be warranted, if only to avoid excessive confusion, multiple re-examinations, and inappropriate treatment. They should not be obtained routinely.

Minimally displaced fractures of the supracondylar region, the condyles, the epicondyles, and the radial head may be difficult to detect in routine radiographic studies. However, periarticular soft tissues may show swelling. Displacement of distal humeral fat pads appears to be related to the extent of intracapsular bleeding. This process, in particular, pushes the dorsal fat pad further posteriorly, so that it becomes more easily evident radiographically.

The majority of epiphyseal injuries are manifested by displacement of the shaft relative to the secondary ossification center, as well as by widening of the growth plate. However, widening of the physis may be extremely difficult to interpret, depending upon the size of the secondary ossification center relative to the entire epiphysis (i.e., the secondary ossification center has not yet formed a definitive subchondral plate). The greater the displacement, the more evident the injury. However, at times, displacement or widening of the plate may be minimal. Epiphyseal injuries occasionally may be seen in only one, not necessarily standard, projection. Rogers reported that 15 to 20% of such injuries were evident only in an oblique view, rather than the standard anteroposterior and lateral views.

If a longitudinal compression force is applied to each end of a naturally curved, tubular bone, the curvature is increased. Up to a certain point, the bone deforms in an elastic manner, and then loses all such deformation once the force is removed. Traumatic bowing of forearm bones or the fibula in children, while not generally recognized as a significant clinical problem, is a definite manifestation of trauma that may occur because of the plastic deformation capacity of developing bones.

Radiopaque, transverse lines across the entire width of the metaphysis in growing long bones may be found in both healthy and sick children (Fig. 5). Usually, transverse lines are distributed relatively symmetrically through the skeleton and occupy identical sites in the corresponding bones on either side of the body. The lines are most evident in the metaphyses that grow most rapidly, such as those of the distal femur and proximal tibia. In the metaphyses of slowest growth, lines may either not form at all or are exceedingly thin. These transverse lines are juxtaposed and parallel to the contours of the physeal provisional zones of calcification. When several transverse lines are present, they tend to parallel one another, each duplicating the contours of the others. The lines nearest the end of the shaft are ordinarily the thickest and widest. Lines farther away from the physis tend to be thinner, less

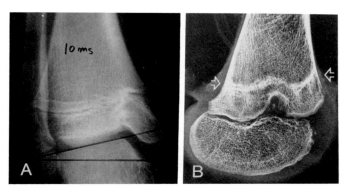

Figure 5. A. Growth slowdown line in the distal tibia demarcates area still undergoing longitudinal growth, in contrast to the nongrowing area with the osseous bridge from metaphysis to medial malleolus. B. Radiograph of distal femur (amputation specimen) showing a transverse growth arrest line (arrows).

distinct, and usually broken and irregular. Within the diaphysis they disappear completely commensurate with endosteal remodeling. Following fracture, the development of a growth slowdown line that does not parallel the physeal contour may be the initial indication of growth plate damage.

Because of difficulty visualizing epiphyseal contours and fractures (Fig. 6), an absolute diagnosis of skeletal injury in children sometimes requires the use of techniques other than routine roentgenography.

STRESS FILMS

Because of the elastic capacity of developing bone and contiguous soft tissues, the injured part often "springs" back into anatomic position after the deforming force is removed. This is particularly common in epiphyseal fractures around the knee. These fractures are the childhood and adolescent analogue of ligamentous injuries in the adult, and one can test for them using similar diagnostic methods. Stress application, may "open" a fracture sufficiently to document the injury (Fig. 7).

ARTHROGRAPHY

This technique probably is more useful in chronic problems than in acute injuries, although it certainly can be used in the latter circumstance (Fig. 8). In infants and young children with suspected epiphyseal fractures of a portion of a radiolucent distal humerus or proximal femur, arthrographic evaluation may allow a correct diagnosis and proper treatment. In the case of chronic problems, arthrographic techniques may make unusual injuries visible.

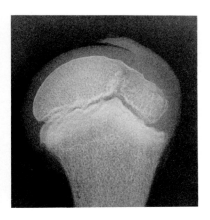

Figure 6.   High intensity contrast film of a specimen of a proximal humerus visualizes the normally radiolucent epiphyseal cartilage.

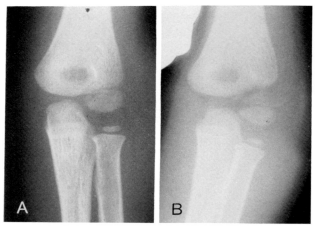

Figure 7. A. Undisplaced fracture of the lateral condyle. B. Stress film defines the instability of the fracture.

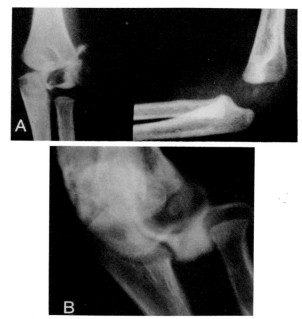

Figure 8. A. Arthrogram outlines a type 3 lateral condylar fracture, which is not readily evident in the lateral view in this infant. B. Arthrogram shows an acute dislocation of the proximal radius.

COMPUTERIZED TOMOGRAPHY

This new technique is particularly useful in the evaluation of spinal trauma. It allows an accurate assessment of narrowing of the spinal canal due to fracture of the posterior or anterior elements, or translation of one vertebra onto the next. It also is the most useful diagnostic method for evaluating fractures of the upper cervical vertebra, a difficult area to assess with routine radiography or standard anteroposterior/lateral tomographic techniques.

SCINTIGRAPHY (RADIONUCLIDE IMAGING)

Systematic application of nuclear medicine procedures probably has been underutilized in children's trauma. The reduced radiation dosage permits repeat and follow-up studies with relative safety. Applications of bone scans include: (1) evaluation of possible fractures in the child with myelodysplasia (Fig. 9); (2) evaluation of radiographically normally appearing bone to detect stress fractures, thus allowing early diagnosis of these lesions; (3) screening for multiple fractures in actual or suspected cases of child abuse; and (4) evaluation of aseptic ischemic necrosis of the capital femoral ossification center following hip dislocation or fracture of the femoral neck.

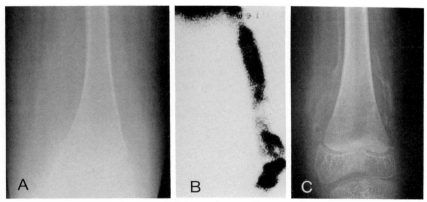

Figure 9. Patient with spina bifida and a swollen, erythematous extremity. A. Roentgenograph of femur on admission. B. Technetium bone scan one day after admission, showing extensive femoral involvement. C. Subperiosteal new bone evident two weeks later. This all was the result of a type 1 injury through the distal femoral physis.

VASCULAR RADIOGRAPHY

While trauma to blood vessels is an infrequent accompaniment to fractures, it represents a potential catastrophe. Fortunately, the increasing awareness of soft-tissue injury and vascular compromise has led to a significant decrease in Volkmann's contracture, whether involving the upper or lower extremity. Arteriography is useful in evaluating complete disruption (Fig. 10), as well as subintimal tears. Venography has less use in childhood and adolescence, since phlebitis and thrombosis are rare complications of chondro-osseous injury prior to skeletal maturation.

MAGNETIC RESONANCE IMAGING

This new technology visualizes cartilaginous and soft-tissue contours much better than other basic studies. However, its expense and limited availability preclude frequent use in the evaluation of most trauma. It undoubtedly will augment or replace CT scans for spinal cord evaluation. Its potential efficacy in evaluating type 3 or 4 growth mechanism fractures remains to be seen. Recent studies by the author have shown that it can be used effectively to delineate osseous bridges forming after growth plate injury and to detect early ischemic changes in the secondary ossification center.

Figure 10. Arteriography demonstrates a complete block in the popliteal artery complicating a type 1 growth mechanism injury of the proximal tibial physis and epiphysis.

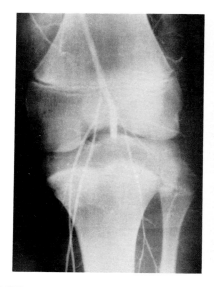

References

Borden S: Roentgen recognition of acute plastic bowing of the forearm in children. Am J Roentgenol 123:524, 1975.

McCarthy SM, Ogden JA: Radiology of postnatal skeletal development: V. Distal humerus. Skel Radiol 7:239, 1982.

McCarthy SM, Ogden JA: Radiology of postnatal skeletal development: VI. Elbow joint, proximal radius and ulna. Skel Radiol 9:17, 1982.

Ogden JA, Conlogue GJ, Jensen P: Radiology of postnatal skeletal development: I. The proximal humerus. Skel Radiol 2:153, 1978.

Ogden JA, Conlogue GJ, Bronson ML: Radiology of postnatal skeletal development: III. The clavicle. Skel Radiol 4:l96, 1979.

Ogden JA, Beall JK, Conlogue GJ, Light TR: Radiology of postnatal skeletal development: IV. Distal radius and ulna. Skel Radiol 6:255, 1981.

Ogden, JA: Radiology of postnatal skeletal development: VIII. Distal tibia and fibula. Skel Radiol 10:209, 1984.

Ogden, JA: Radiology of postnatal skeletal development: IX. Proximal tibia and fibula. Skel Radiol 11:169, 1984.

Ogden JA: Radiology of postnatal skeletal development: X. Patella and tibial tuberosity. Skel Radiol 11:246, 1984.

Ogden JA: Growth slowdown and arrest lines. J Ped Orthop 4:409, 1984.

Rogers LF: The radiography of epiphyseal injuries. Am J Roentgenol 96:289, 1970.

Silverman, FN (ed): Caffey's Pediatric X-ray Diagnosis: An Integrated Imaging Approach (8th ed). Chicago: Yearbook Med Publ, 1985.

Growth Mechanism Injury—General Aspects

Approximately 15% of all fractures in children involve the physis (growth plate). Boys sustain physeal injuries more frequently than girls. Undoubtedly this occurs because of the greater exposure of boys to significant etiologic factors, especially uncontrolled and controlled trauma from athletic activities. Further, the physes stay open longer in boys than in girls, extending the duration of exposure to potential injury. There also may be intrinsic response differences during the growth spurt. The distal physes are injured more commonly than the proximal physes. This high incidence of injury to certain physes, such as the distal radius, distal tibia, and phalanges, may result from increased exposure of these more distal regions to trauma, rather than from any unique physiologic susceptibility of these particular physes.

IN ANY INJURY TO A GROWTH MECHANISM, NO MATTER HOW MINOR IT MAY APPEAR, IT IS IMPERATIVE THAT THE RISK OF GROWTH SLOWDOWN OR ARREST, SHORTENING, AND ANGULAR DEFORMITY BE DISCUSSED WITH THE PARENTS.

References

Bright RW: Physeal injuries. In Rockwood CA, Wilkins KE, King RE (eds): Fractures: Children (Vol 3). Philadelphia, JB Lippincott, 1984.

Grogan DP, Ogden JA: Letter to the editor: "Thurstan Holland fragment." J Bone Joint Surg 67-A:980, 1985.

Ogden JA: Injury to the growth mechanism of the immature skeleton. Skel Radiol 6:237, 1981.

Ogden JA: Skeletal growth mechanism injury patterns. J Ped Orthop 2:371–377, 1982.

Salter RB, Harris WR: Injuries involving epiphyseal plates. J Bone Joint Surg 45A:587, 1963.

Growth Mechanism Injury—General Aspects Type 1

Figures 11–13

Anatomy

-The fracture extends transversely across the hypertrophic and calcified zones of the physis
-Microscopic undulation varies and may involve the germinal zones
-Displacement may be minimal, making this pattern hard to diagnose radiographically

Clinical Considerations

-This is the most common injury pattern in infants and young children
-It must be strongly considered, instead of dislocations, which are anatomically less likely
-This pattern is frequent in child abuse and myelomeningocele patients

Treatment

-Closed reduction is indicated for most type 1 injuries
-Gentle reduction with adequate anesthesia (not amnesia) minimizes microscopic trauma when the displaced physis and epiphysis are placed back on the metaphysis
-Infrequently, open reduction may be necessary
-In certain injuries, such as the distal humerus in infants, and young children, temporary pin fixation may be necessary

Complications

-Most of these injuries heal uneventfully
-However, the pattern may be associated with growth slowdown or arrest, especially when areas such as the distal ulna or proximal radius are involved

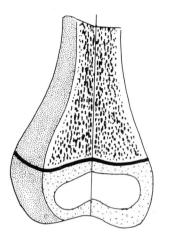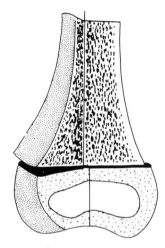

Figure 11. Schematic of a normal epiphysis and physis and a minimally displaced type 1 injury.

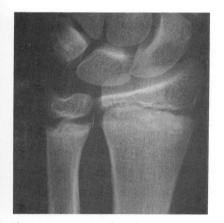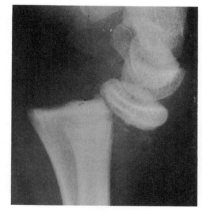

Figure 12. Typical undisplaced type 1 injuries of the distal radius and ulna.

Figure 13. Displaced type 1 injury of the distal radius.

Growth Mechanism Injury—General Aspects Type 2

Anatomy

-The fracture extends partially along the physeal-metaphyseal interface, and then propagates into the metaphysis, creating the characteristic triangular fragment (Thurstan Holland sign)

-This metaphyseal fragment varies in size, and may require special views (e.g., oblique) to verify its presence

Clinical Considerations

-This is the most common injury pattern, becoming increasingly prevalent after four years

Treatment

-Closed reduction is usually indicated

-Reduction must be done *gently*

-The periosteum is intact along the metaphyseal fragment and diaphysis, creating a stable hinge to "work against" during reduction

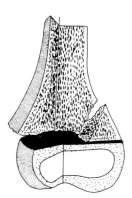

Figure 14. Schematic of the type 2 injury pattern.

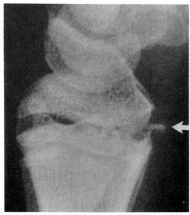

Figure 15. Type 2 injury of the distal radius (arrow) showing a small metaphyseal fragment (Thurstan Holland sign).

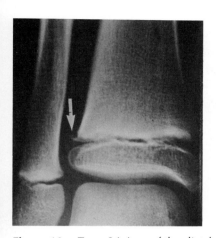

Figure 16. Type 2 injury of the distal tibia showing a small metaphyseal fragment (arrow) only evident in the mortise view.

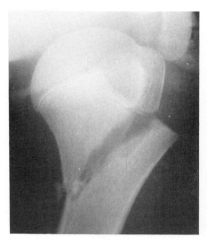

Figure 17. Type 2 injury of the proximal humerus showing a large metaphyseal fragment.

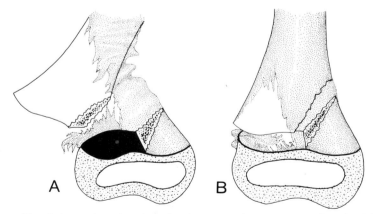

Figure 18. Schematics showing the intact periosteum associated with the metaphyseal fragment (A), and how this tissue sleeve imparts some stability during reduction (B).

-Infrequently, open reduction may be necessary, especially to remove soft tissues displaced into the fracture gap
-Internal fixation is rarely necessary, even if open reduction is undertaken (usually the shaft buttonholes through the periosteum)

Complications
-Most type 2 injuries heal without significant consequences
-The major long-term problems are growth slowdown or arrest, which may be localized, leading to an angular deformity, or complete, leading to a length inequality (especially when the distal femur is involved)

Growth Mechanism Injury—General Aspects Type 3

Anatomy
-The fracture propagates transversely along the physeal-metaphyseal interface and then turns to cross the entire physis, epiphysis, ossification center, and articular cartilage
-This creates an unstable epiphyseal fragment with disruption of *all* zones of the growth plate and loss of continuity of the articular surface

Treatment
-These injuries invariably require open reduction and internal fixation
-Particular attention must be directed at restoration of the articular surfaces
-Whenever possible, fixation pins or screws should be placed transversely, going from the disrupted epiphyseal fragment to the uninjured epiphysis, rather than crossing the physis

Complications
-Growth arrest
-Angulation deformity
-Longitudinal growth deformity
-Articular deformity
-Non-union

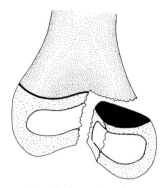

Figure 19. Schematic of type 3 injury.

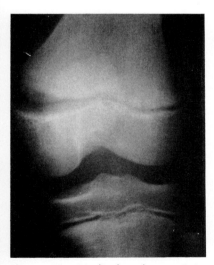

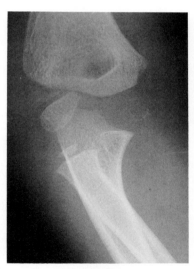

Figure 20. Undisplaced type 3 injury of the distal femur which was made evident by a stress film, causing medial widening of the physis. Minimally displaced injuries must be watched extremely closely, since increasing displacement may occur as the soft tissue swelling subsides.

Figure 21. Displaced type 3 injury of the distal humerus (lateral condyle).

Growth Mechanism Injury—General Aspects Type 4

Figures 22–26

Anatomy

-The fracture extends from the articular surface to the metaphyseal cortex, traversing epiphysis (and its ossification center), physis, and metaphyseal bone
-The metaphyseal fragments of type 2 and type 4 injuries may be confusing. However, the treating physician must distinguish between them to institute proper treatment

Treatment

-Requires open reduction and internal fixation
-Both the physis and articular surface must be anatomically restored
-As in type 3 patterns, fixation devices should be directed transversely, whenever feasible

Complications

-Growth arrest
-Angulation deformity
-Longitudinal growth deformity
-Articular deformity

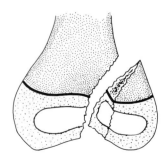

Figure 22. Schematic of type 4 injury.

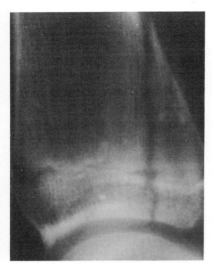

Figure 23. Tomogram of undis-placed type 4 injury of the posterior malleolus of the distal tibia.

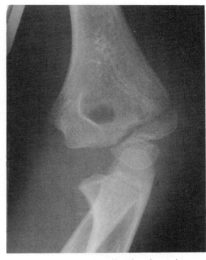

Figure 24. Minimally displaced type 4 injury of the distal humerus (lateral condyle).

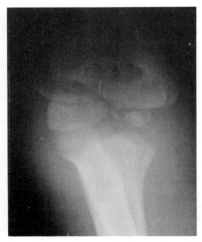

Figure 25. Delayed union of type 4 lateral condyle fracture. Displace-ment of the condylar fragment oc-curred while the patient was immo-bilized.

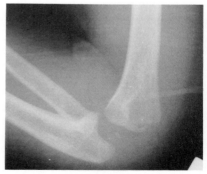

Figure 26. Apparent type 4 lateral condyle injury was really a type 2 separation of the entire distal hu-merus.

Growth Mechanism Injury—General Aspects Type 5

Anatomy

-Originally felt to be due to a crushing of the physis
-Microscopic splitting, linear disruption, and microvascular compromise of the physis are more likely mechanisms

Clinical Considerations

-Controversial pattern which cannot be diagnosed at the original time of injury
-This diagnosis usually is made retrospectively

Treatment

-If suspected, three to four weeks of nonweight bearing (lower extremity) or immobilization (upper extremity)
-Serial follow-up roentgenography

Complications

-Longitudinal growth slowdown or arrest
-Angular deformity
-Shortening of arm or leg

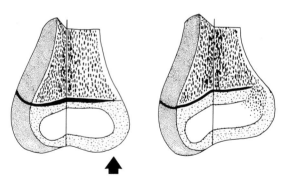

Figure 27. Schematic of type 5 injury (left) leading to angular growth deformity (right).

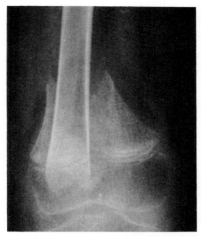

Figure 28. Central type 5 injury in a myelomeningocoele patient who stood on his leg after eight weeks in a hip spica and impacted his distal femoral metaphysis into the epiphysis.

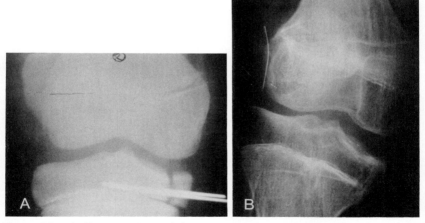

Figure 29. A. Type 3 injury of the proximal tibia without any other obvious injury. This was treated with an open reduction and pin fixation. B. Follow-up showed not only growth arrest of the type 3 proximal tibial injury (despite anatomic reduction and fixation) but a medial growth arrest of the distal femur, leading to angular deformity.

Growth Mechanism Injury—General Aspects Type 6

Figures 30–31

Anatomy
-Involves the peripheral region of the growth plate, particularly the zone of Ranvier
-May not always be associated with a major fracture
-Usually results from a localized contusion or avulsion of the peripheral portion of the growth mechanism concerned specifically with latitudinal or appositional cartilaginous growth

Clinical Considerations
-May result from a glancing type of trauma involving avulsion of overlying skin and subcutaneous tissues, such as might occur from a lawn mower, from extension of a traumatically induced infection or severe burn, or if the ankle is caught in a spoked bicycle wheel

Treatment
-Local care of soft tissue injury
-Do *not* replace small avulsion fragments
-Reduction of large fragments
-Frequent follow-up

Complications
-Peripheral osseous bridge formation frequently occurs, and leads to peripherally localized epiphysiodesis
-Progressive angular deformity
-This bridge is frequently amenable to surgical resection

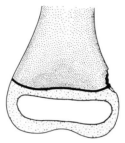

Figure 30.   Schematic of type 6 injury pattern.

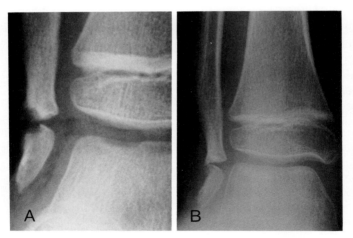

Figure 31.   A. Type 6 injury of the distal fibula from a lawn mower. B. Beginning bridge formation and angular deformity several months later.

Growth Mechanism Injury—General Aspects Type 7

Anatomy

-Completely intraepiphyseal fracture propagating from the articular surface through the epiphyseal cartilage into or adjacent to the secondary ossification center
-Does not involve the primary physis
-May affect the smaller "physis" around the secondary center of ossification
-Common at the malleoli, within the distal humerus (capitellum) or distal femur as an osteochondral fracture, and in the tibial tuberosity (Osgood-Schlatter lesion)

Treatment

-Immobilization when undisplaced
-Open reduction and fixation when displaced

Complications

-Non-union
-Displacement into joint (loose body)
-Articular surface changes
-Chronic synovitis or effusion
-Chronic pain

38   POCKET GUIDE TO PEDIATRIC FRACTURES

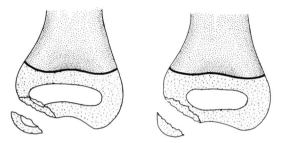

Figure 32. Schematic of type 7 injuries.

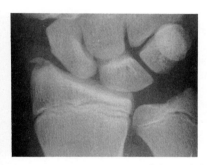

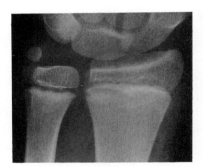

Figure 33. Type 7 injury of the radial styloid.

Figure 34. Radiographic non-union of type 7 injury of the ulnar styloid accompanying a type 1 distal radial fracture (healed).

Growth Mechanism Injury—General Aspects Type 8

Anatomy

-Involves the metaphyseal growth and remodeling mechanisms
-Represents temporary phenomenon related to vascular alterations
-The metaphyseal circulation involved in formation of primary spongiosa from the cartilage cell columns is temporarily disrupted, leading to failure of normal osseous remodeling and subsequent, transiently increased osseous density and physeal widening

Treatment

-Appropriate reduction and immobilization for the area involved

Complications

-Following rapid revascularization, the junction of primary spongiosa and hypertrophic cartilage may become biomechanically weaker, not unlike the revascularization phase of Legg-Perthes disease
-Epiphysiolysis may be a complication of this temporary metaphyseal ischemia
-Hypervascularity may lead to angular growth (e.g., tibia valgus complicating proximal metaphyseal fracture)

Type 8

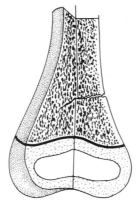

Figure 35. Schematic of type 8 injury.

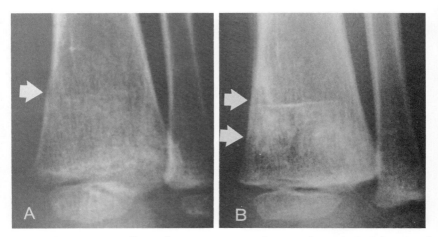

Figure 36. A. Minimally evident acute type 8 fracture (arrow). B. Sclerosis of bone due to temporary ischemia occurs at the fracture line and between it and the physis (arrows). The remainder of well-vascularized bone between the nutrient foramen and fracture line undergoes a relative disuse osteoporosis from lack of weight-bearing.

Growth Mechanism Injury—General Aspects Type 9

Anatomy

-Involves the diaphyseal growth mechanism of appositional, membranous bone formation from the periosteum
-Any direct injury causing permanent damage to the periosteum may affect the ability of the bone to increase cortical volume circumferentially

Clinical Considerations

-May be associated with severe fragmentation of portions of the diaphysis, which is a significant problem if the damaged bone requires a thick diaphyseal cortex for normal biomechanical function (e.g., tibia)
-The periosteum may be damaged in a localized area, which may lead to unusual patterns of extraperiosteal bone formation
-Wringer injuries may be associated with significant avulsion of the periosteum
-Damage to the interosseous area in paired bones also may cause contiguity of damaged periosteal elements, leading to synostosis

Treatment

-Evaluate muscle compartment pressures
-Appropriate care of soft tissues
-Stabilization of fracture fragments by either open or closed methods

Complications

-Non-union with pain
-Synostosis

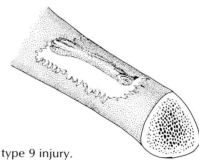

Figure 37.   Schematic of type 9 injury.

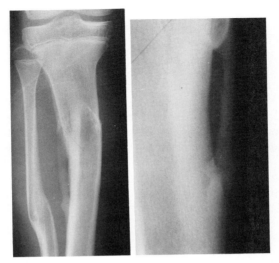

Figure 38. A. Type 9 tibial lesion. B. Oblique view showing separation from the tibia and a pseudarthrosis at the distal end.

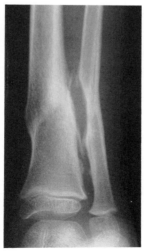

Figure 39. Synostosis following tibia/fibula fracture. This is recurring four months after an initial attempt at resection.

Neonatal Fractures

Figure 40

-Usually the result of a traumatic or difficult delivery
-Most common diaphyseal fracture is the clavicle
-Evaluate for dysplastic or metabolic abnormality
-Epiphyseal injuries easy to confuse with dislocation
-Most common epiphyseal injuries involve the shoulder (proximal humerus), elbow (distal humerus), and hip (proximal femur)
-Spinal cord may be injured without actual fracture of the spine

References

Gresham EL: Birth trauma. Pediatr Clin North Am 22:317, 1975.
Koch BM, Eng GM: Neonatal spinal cord injury. Arch Phys Med Rehab 60:378, 1979.

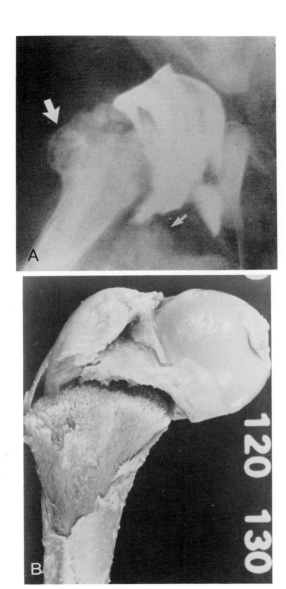

Figure 40. A. Birth fracture of entire proximal femoral epiphysis (easy to confuse with dislocation). B. Specimen of proximal femur from a stillborn demonstrating the proximal femoral fracture and periosteal stripping.

Myelodysplasia

Figures 41–43

-Disuse atrophy makes diaphysis and metaphyses extremely susceptible to compression injury
-Always consider as part of evaluation of fever of unknown origin in such a child (see Fig. 9 for use of bone scan)
-Lack of knowledge on child's part may lead to massive callus formation due to chronic motion and extensive periosteal stripping, especially when a physeal fracture occurs

Reference

Wenger DR, Jeffcoat BT, Herring JA: The guarded prognosis of physeal injury in paraplegic children. J Bone Joint Surg 62:241, 1980.

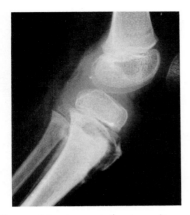

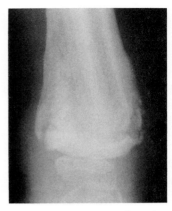

Figure 41. Lucent fracture line of acute proximal tibial type 1 injury in a myelodysplastic patient.

Figure 42. Excessive callus due to chronic motion of a type 1 injury of the distal tibia in a myelodysplastic patient.

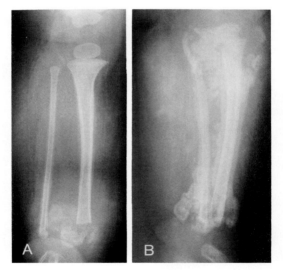

Figure 43. Excessive bone formation following epiphyseolysis complicating corrective clubfoot surgery in a myelodysplastic patient. A. Three weeks after surgery. There is considerable callus from a distal tibial epiphyseolysis. However, notice a small metaphyseal fracture at the medial proximal tibia. B. Six weeks after surgery, proximal callus is now readily evident.

Osteogenesis Imperfecta Figure 44

-Several varieties of severity
-Must be treated as soon as possible to minimize progressive deformation
-Can lead to severe deformities
-Necessity of multiple level osteotomies

Reference

Mitchell OC: Fractures in brittle bone diseases. Orthop Clin North Am 3:787, 1972.

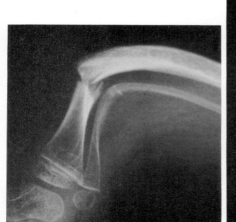
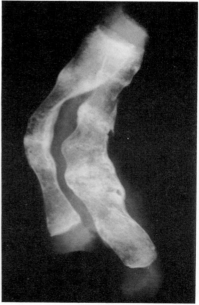

Figure 44: A. Typical bowing of tibia and fibula with apical fracture in a child with osteogenesis imperfecta. B. Multiple fractures of the radius and ulna in a fatal case of osteogenesis imperfecta.

Head Injury

Figure 45

-Major complication is inability to control fractures due to decerebrate
 rigidity
-Open reduction and internal fixation often indicated
-Alternatively, external fixators may be temporarily useful
-Heterotopic bone around joint is a common complication

Reference

Hoffer M, Garrett A, Brink J: The orthopaedic management of brain injured children. J
    Bone Joint Surg 53-A:567, 1971.

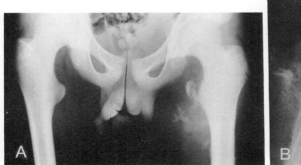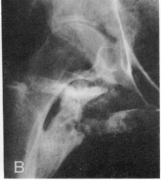

Figure 45.   A. Early heterotopic bone formation around the left lesser trochanter in a head-injured teenager. B. Massive heterotopic bone in a 16-year-old
girl three years after recovery from a closed head injury (approximately seven
weeks of decerebrate rigidity and coma).

Stress Fractures Figure 46

-May be confused with neoplasms if seen early
-Often present when new sport attempted, or too much activity in a
 regular sport
-Fibula and tibula most common sites
-May affect medial proximal tibia, as in adult
-Many osteochondroses (e.g., Panner's, Sever's and Osgood-Schlatter's
 disease) may be examples of chronic overuse injuries to epiphyses
 from childhood sports

References

Devas MB: Stress fractures in children. J Bone Joint Surg 45B:528, 1963.
Engh CA, Robinson RA, Milgram J: Stress fractures in children. J Trauma 10:532, 1970.

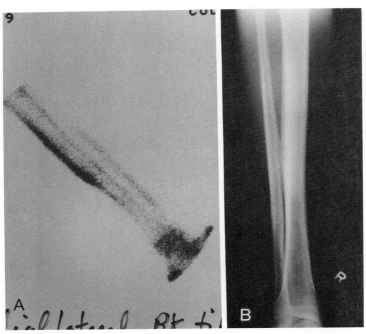

Figure 46. A. Positive bone scan in 14-year-old jogger. B. Tibial subperiosteal bone evident several weeks later.

Child Abuse

Figure 47–48

-Characteristic peripheral lesion
-Multiple fractures in different stages of healing
-Necessity for coordination with pediatric staff and state regulatory
 agencies

References

Akbarnia CH, Akbarnia NO: The role of the orthopaedist in child abuse and neglect. Orthop Clin North Amer 7:733, 1976.

Kempe CH, Helfer RE (eds): The Battered Child. Chicago, Univ. of Chicago Press, 1980.

Kleinman, PK, Marks SC, Blackbourne B: The metaphyseal lesion in abused infants: a radiologic-histopathologic study. Am J Roent 146:895, 1986.

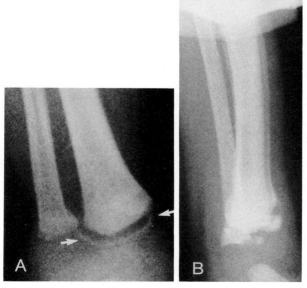

Figure 47. A. Child abuse fracture of the distal tibia. This thin linear fracture (arrows) would be a small triangle in the lateral, much like the proximal tibial injury in Fig. 43A. B. Distal tibial injury from child abuse showing extensive subperiosteal new bone formation from periosteal stripping.

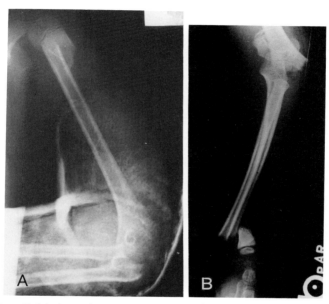

Figure 48. Child abuse fractures occurring after this three-year-old child was thrown from a porch. A. Proximal humeral injury. B. Concomitant distal humeral and distal radioulnar fractures.

Clavicle
Proximal

Anatomy
-A physis and epiphysis are present, along with a meniscus and soft
  tissue continuity with the sternum
-True sternoclavicular dislocation is very unlikely prior to 20 years
-Instead, a physeal injury (type 1 or 2) occurs

Clinical Diagnosis
-Pain over sternoclavicular joint
-If anteriorly displaced, the proximal end is palpable
-If posteriorly displaced, a "hollow" is evident, and there may be
  difficulty swallowing or breathing

Radiologic Diagnosis
-Oblique sternoclavicular joint views
-Cross-sectional imaging

Recommended Treatment
-Attempt closed reduction for anterior displacement
-May require pin fixation to ensure stability
-Posterior displacement usually requires open reduction

Complications
-Protrusion into mediastinal structures
-Tracheal or esophageal pressure
-Chronic pain if left unreduced

Reference
Brooks A, Henning G.: Injury to the proximal clavicular epiphysis. J Bone Joint Surg 54-
    A1347, 1972.

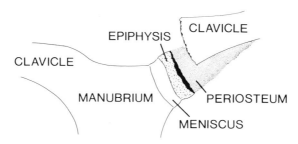

Figure 49. Schematic of injury pattern to the proximal clavicular physis. The epiphysis remains attached to the sternum (manubrium).

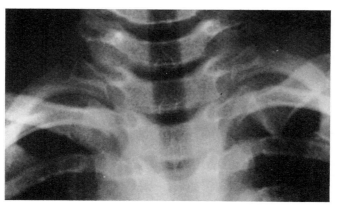

Figure 50. Radiograph of left proximal clavicular fracture in a four-year-old.

Clavicle Diaphysis

Figures 51–53

Anatomy
-Tend to be within the major curve
-Do not confuse with congenital pseudarthrosis

Clinical Diagnosis
-Most common fracture in the preschool child
-Palpable deformity
-Angulation common (watch for skin injury)

Radiologic Diagnosis
-Comminution more likely in older children
-Greenstick pattern common
-Abundant callus formation

Recommended Treatment
-Accurate anatomic reduction rarely necessary
-Figure of eight clavicle strap; may require readjustments during first seven to ten days

Complications
-Children under three years of age tend to get massive callus but this remodels (usually within a year)
-Neurovascular complications unusual
-Permanent angular deformity uncommon

Reference

Calandi C, Bartolozzi G: On 110 cases of fracture of the clavicle in the newborn. Clin Pediatr 64:541, 1959.

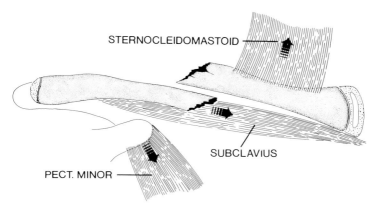

Figure 51. Schematic of displaced, overriding fracture of the diaphysis of the clavicle.

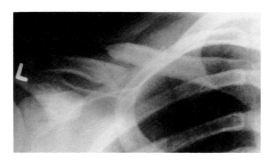

Figure 52. Roentgenograph of fracture of the clavicle in a six-year-old.

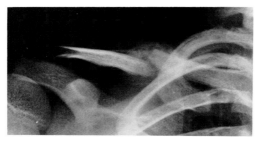

Figure 53. Rapid, abundant callus formation one month after clavicular fracture in a nine-year-old.

Clavicle
Distal

Anatomy
-Usually a type 1 or type 2 physeal injury
-*Not* a true joint dislocation prior to skeletal maturity
-Periosteal sleeve partially intact and attached to intact acromioclavicular joint

Clinical Diagnosis
-Painful over acromioclavicular joint
-Easy to confuse with acromioclavicular separation
-Distal end of clavicle may be prominent, depending upon extent of separation

Radiologic Diagnosis
-Easy to confuse with acromioclavicular separation
-May require stress view (have patient hold weight)

Recommended Treatment
-Closed reduction
-Internal fixation (percutaneous) if unstable

Complications
-Excessive subperiosteal bone which, in the extreme, may create a "second" distal clavicle

References
Ogden JA: Distal clavicular physeal injury. Clin Orthop 188:68–73, 1984.
Rockwood CA: Fractures of the outer clavicle in children and adults. J Bone Joint Surg 64B:642, 1982.

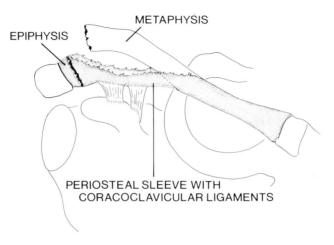

EPIPHYSIS

METAPHYSIS

PERIOSTEAL SLEEVE WITH
CORACOCLAVICULAR LIGAMENTS

Figure 54. Schematic of a distal clavicular injury.

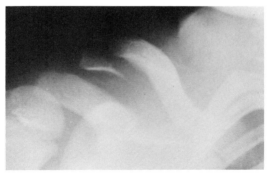

Figure 55. Radiograph showing similarity to an acromioclavicular separation in a young adult, with downward displacement of the shoulder. However, the acromioclavicular joint is intact.

Shoulder Dislocation

Figures 56–57

Anatomy
-Neonate does *not* dislocate (physeal fracture of the proximal humerus instead)
-Unusual injury prior to skeletal maturity

Clinical Diagnosis
-Loss of motion
-Palpable gap under acromion

Radiologic Diagnosis
-Displacement of humerus from glenoid

Treatment
-Closed reduction

Complication
-Recurrent dislocation
-Child may be able to habitually duplicate the dislocation

Reference

Wagner KT, Lyne ED: Adolescent traumatic dislocations of the shoulder with open epiphysis. J Pediatr Orthop 3:60, 1983.

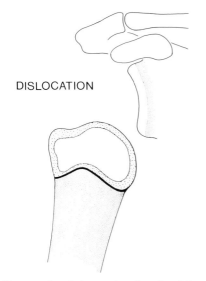

DISLOCATION

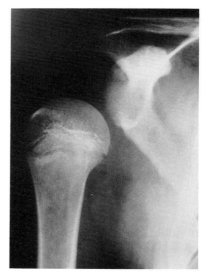

Figure 56. Schematic of a shoulder dislocation.

Figure 57. Radiographic appearance of a shoulder dislocation in a ten-year-old.

Humerus
Proximal Epiphysis

Anatomy
-Changing physeal contour from transverse to pyramidal
-Type 1 injury common under ten years
-Type 2 pattern common over ten years

Clinical Diagnosis
-Painful shoulder
-Laterally displaced metaphysis may be palpable

Radiologic Diagnosis
-Epiphyseal and metaphyseal fragments usually medially displaced
-May be shortening (overriding) in younger child
-Often misinterpreted as shoulder dislocation in neonate following difficult delivery

Recommended Treatment
-Closed reduction, followed by appropriate immobilization (sling and swathe or cast)
-Avoid "Statue of Liberty" cast
-Bed rest with arm in abduction, if unstable
-Internal fixation rarely indicated
-Overriding acceptable, except in patient approaching skeletal maturity

Complications
-Longitudinal growth slowdown
-Humerus varus
-Herniation through periosteal sleeve
-Entrapment of biceps tendon

References

Kohler R, Trillaut JM: Fracture and fracture separation of the proximal humerus in children: report of 136 cases. J Pediatr Orthop 3:326–332, 1983
Lemperg R, Lilliequist B: Dislocation of the proximal epiphysis of the humerus in newborns. Acta Paediatr Scand 59:377–380, 1970.

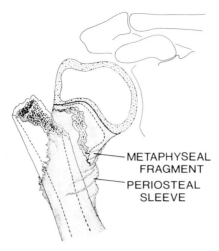

METAPHYSEAL
FRAGMENT

PERIOSTEAL
SLEEVE

Figure 58. Schematic of injury to the proximal humeral physis and epiphysis, showing herniation of lateral metaphysis through a rent in the periosteal sleeve.

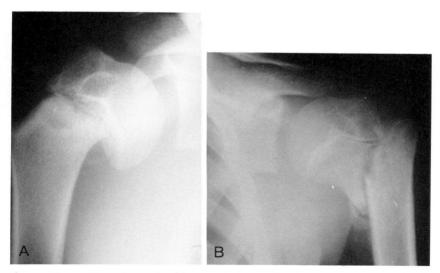

Figure 59. A. Type 1 proximal humeral physeal fracture in seven-year-old. B. Type 2 proximal humeral fracture in a 12-year-old showing the lateral and superior displacement of the metaphysis. This amount of shortening usually will correct by skeletal maturation.

Humerus
Proximal Metaphysis

Figures 60–62

Anatomy
-Similar to epiphyseal injury

Clinical Diagnosis
-Shoulder pain

Radiologic Diagnosis
-Greenstick or torus injury common

Recommended Treatment
-Closed reduction, when necessary, followed by sling and swathe
-1–2 cm overriding acceptable

Complications
-Unusual
-Longitudinal overgrowth may occur

Reference

Nilsson S, Svartholm F: Fracture of the upper end of humerus in children. Acta Chir Scand 130:433–439, 1965.

PROXIMAL METAPHYSIS

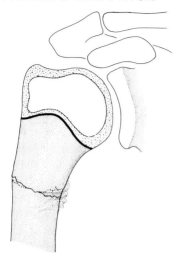

Figure 60. Schematic of injury to the proximal humeral metaphysis.

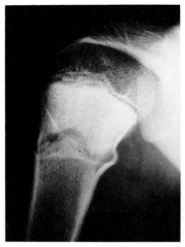

Figure 61. Typical undisplaced torus fracture of the proximal humeral metaphysis.

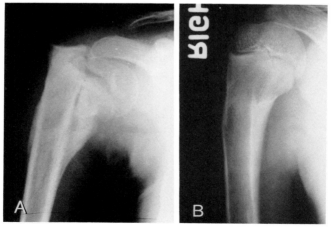

Figure 62. A. Roentgenogram of displaced and overriding metaphyseal fracture in a five-year-old victim of child abuse. B. Four years later the injury has extensively remodeled.

Humerus Diaphysis

Anatomy
-Cortex is progressively rigid, leading to changing patterns of fracture

Clinical Diagnosis
-Angular deformity, swelling

Radiologic Diagnosis
-Greenstick injury common
-Spiral fracture in adolescent
-May displace when complete

Recommended Treatment
-Closed reduction

Complications
-Radial nerve injury
-Longitudinal overgrowth
-Angulation

Reference

Holm CL: Management of humeral shaft fractures. Fundamental nonoperative techniques. Clin Orthop 71:132–139, 1970.

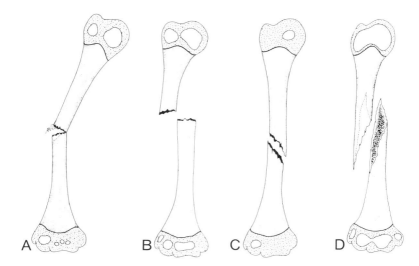

Figure 63. Schematic showing undisplaced or greenstick (A), transverse (B), oblique (C), and spiral (D) patterns of humeral diaphyseal fractures.

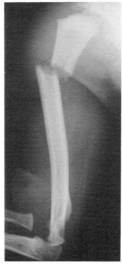

Figure 64. Radiograph of a partially displaced diaphyseal fracture in a six-year-old.

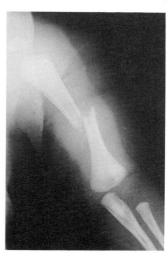

Figure 65. Displaced fracture of the humerus due to traumatic delivery.

Humerus
Supracondylar
(Distal Metaphysis)

Figures 66–70

Anatomy
-Double column due to olecranon and coronoid fossae, making reductions unstable

Clinical Diagnosis
-Swollen elbow
-Detailed neurovascular assessment essential

Radiologic Diagnosis
-Usually posterior displacement with extensive periosteal stripping
-*Beware*: impacted fracture may be in varus when undisplaced

Recommended Treatment
-Initial closed reduction, with or without percutaneous pinning
-Skeletal traction
-Open reduction

Complications
-Nerve injury
-Vascular injury
-Compartment syndrome
-Cubitus varus
-Physeal injury

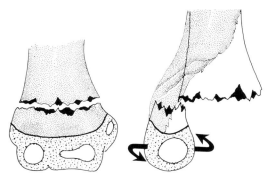

Figure 66. Schematics of undisplaced (left) and displaced, rotated (left) supra-condylar fractures of the distal humerus.

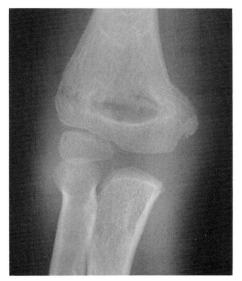

Figure 67. Typical undisplaced fracture, impacted in varus.

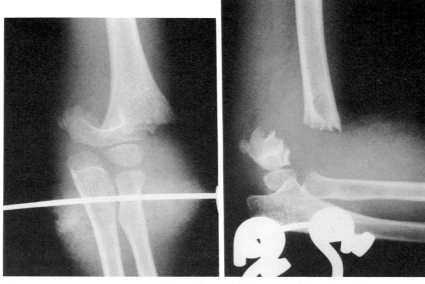

Figure 68. Anteroposterior (A) and lateral (B) views of displaced fracture just after placement in olecranon traction.

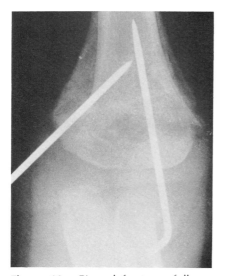

Figure 69. Pinned fracture, following open reduction.

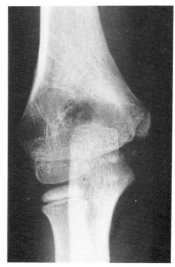

Figure 70. Varus complication one year after injury.

References

Labell H, Bunnell WB, Duhaime M, Poitras B: Cubitus varus deformity following supra-condylar fractures of the humerus in children. J Pediatr Orthop 3:539–546, 1982.

Oppenheim WL, Clader TJ, Smith C, Bayer M: Supracondylar humeral osteotomy for traumatic childhood cubitus varus deformity. Clin Orthop l88:34–39, 1984.

Rowell PJW: Arterial occlusion in juvenile humeral supracondylar fracture. Injury 6:254–256, 1974.

Humerus Transcondylar (Physeal)

Anatomy
-Usually a type 1 injury, especially in the neonate

Clinical Diagnosis
-Must be distinguished from elbow dislocation
-Frequent as birth injury

Radiologic Diagnosis
-Usually medially displaced (whereas a dislocation is usually laterally displaced)

Recommended Treatment
-Closed reduction
-Open reduction and fixation

Complications
-Angular deformity, similar to supracondylar fracture (cubitus varus)

References

DeLee JC, Wilkins KE, Rogers, LF, Rockwood, CA: Fracture separation of the distal humeral epiphysis. J Bone Joint Surg 62A:46–51, 1980.

Holda ME, Monole A, LaMont RL: Epiphyseal separations of the distal end of the humerus with medial displacement. J Bone Joint Surg 52A:52–57, 1980.

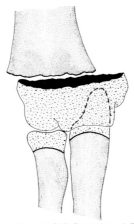

TRANSCONDYLAR

Figure 71. Schematic of a distal humeral transcondylar fracture.

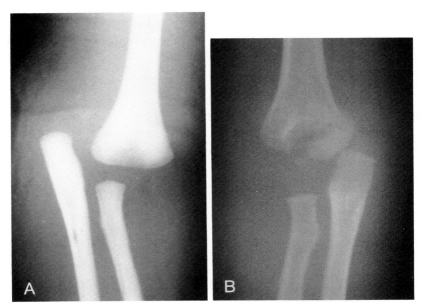

Figure 72. A. Type 1 transcondylar fracture of the distal humerus in a newborn. This must be distinguished from an elbow dislocation. The ulna usually is more centrally located relative to the distal humerus. B. Type 2 transcondylar fracture in a three-month-old following child abuse.

Humerus
Lateral Condylar

Anatomy
-Type 3 or 4 physeal/epiphyseal injury

Clinical Diagnosis
-Pain, swelling
-May also have soft tissue damage medially

Radiologic Diagnosis
-Assess degree of displacement
-Stress film may be indicated (see Fig. 5)

Recommended Treatment
-Pin fixation, with open reduction in most cases
-Beware the undisplaced or minimally displaced injury: reassess within
 a few days, and alter treatment as necessary

Complications
-Loss of reduction after a few days when swelling subsides
-Relative instability of "undisplaced lesion"
-Delayed union
-Non-union
-Avascular necrosis
-Premature physeal closure
-Valgus deformity (static or progressive)
-Delayed ulnar nerve damage

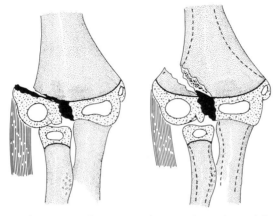

Figure 73. Schematics of type 3 and type 4 lateral condylar fractures.

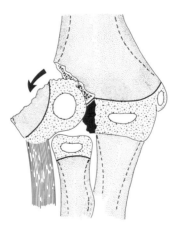

Figure 74. Schematic of rotation of lateral condylar fragment due to muscle pull from the common extensor origins.

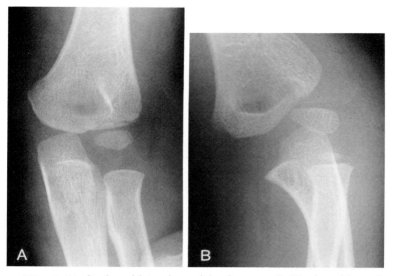

Figure 75. A. Undisplaced lateral condylar fracture. B. Displaced lateral condylar fracture.

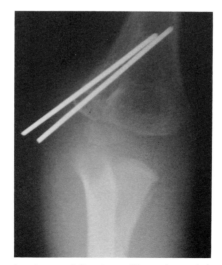

Figure 76. Open reduction and fixation of lateral condylar fracture.

References

Flynn JC, Richards JF: Non-union of minimally displaced fractures of the lateral condyle of the humerus in children. J Bone Joint Surg 53:1096–1101, 1971.

Hardacre JA, Nahigian SH, Froimson AI, Brown JE: Fracture of the lateral condyle of the humerus in children. J Bone Joint Surg 53-A:1083–1095, 1971.

Jakob R, Fowles JV, Rang, M, Kassib MT: Observations concerning fractures of the lateral humeral condyle in children. J Bone Joint Surg 57B:430–436, 1975.

Humerus
Medial Condyle

Anatomy
-Type 3 or 4 physeal/epiphyseal injury

Clinical Diagnosis
-Swollen, painful elbow

Radiologic Diagnosis
-Usually displaced
-May be part of "T" intercondylar fractures
-May be confused with medial epicondylar fracture

Recommended Treatment
-Open reduction, internal fixation

Complications
-Delayed union
-Non-union
-"Fishtail" deformity

References

Fahey JJ, O'Brien ET: Fracture separation of the medial humeral condyle in a child confused with fracture of the medial epicondyle. J Bone Joint Surg 53A:1102–1104, 1971.

Fowles JV, Kassab MT: Displaced fractures in the medial humeral condyle in children. J Bone Joint Surg 53A:1102–1104, 1971.

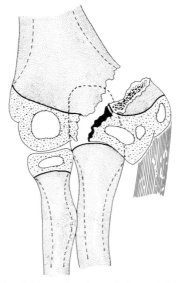

Figure 77. Schematic of medial condylar fracture.

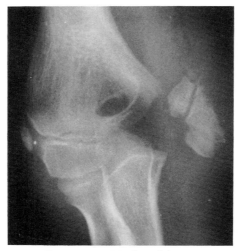

Figure 78. Displaced fracture.

Humerus
Lateral Epicondyle

Figure 79

Anatomy
-Major muscular attachment
-Nonarticular injury

Clinical Diagnosis
-Very infrequent injury

Radiologic Diagnosis
-Displacement varies
-Comparison views usually unnecessary

Treatment
-Closed if only 1 to 2 mm displacement (must be reassessed within a
 few days to evaluate change in displacement
-Open reduction with fixation

Complications
-Delayed union
-Non-union
-Elbow instability

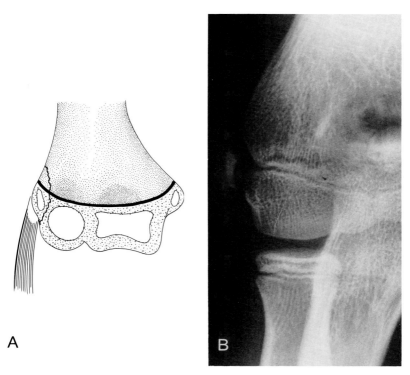

Figure 79. A. Schematic of lateral epicondylar fracture. B. Radiograph of injury—minimal displacement.

Humerus
Medial Epicondyle

Anatomy
-Major muscular attachment
-May displace progressively due to isometric contractures

Clinical Diagnosis

-May be part of elbow dislocation (the epicondyle may be within the joint)

Radiologic Diagnosis
-Displacement varies, and may change (worsen) over several days as the soft tissue swelling decreases
-Stress films may be necessary to assess *real* extent of displacement

Treatment
-Closed if separation minimal (less than 2 mm)
-Pin fixation and open reduction
-Neurolysis of cubital tunnel and ulnar nerve

Complications
-Ulnar nerve injury (acute or chronic)
-Delayed union
-Non-union
-Chronic pain
-Elbow instability

References

Bernstein SM, King JD, Sanderson RA: Fractures of the medial epicondyle of the humerus. Contemp Orthop 3:637–641, 1981.

Woods GM, Tullos HG: Elbow instability and medial epicondyle fracture. Am J Sports Med 5:23–30, 1977.

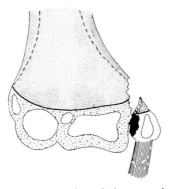

Figure 80. Schematic of medial epicondylar fracture.

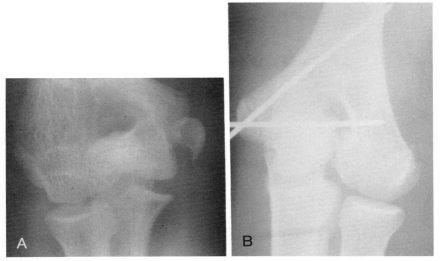

Figure 81. A. Displaced medial epicondylar fracture. B. Open reduction and pinning of medial epicondylar fracture.

Elbow
"Little League Elbow"

Anatomy

-Sometimes referred to as Panner's disease
-Osteochondritis of capitellum

Clinical Diagnosis

-Pain in elbow especially when throwing

Radiologic Diagnosis

-Sclerotic and lytic regions
-Technetium bone scan

Recommended Treatment

-Discontinue sports
-Switch to different position in sport
-Change daily time commitment to sport
-Immobilization

Complications

-Joint incongruency
-Loss of motion

Reference

Roberts N, Hughes R: Osteochondritis dissecans of the elbow joint. A clinical study. J Bone Joint Surg 32-B:348, 1950.

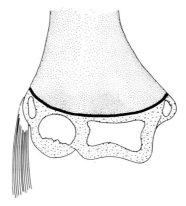

Figure 82. Schematic of damage to the capitellar ossification center.

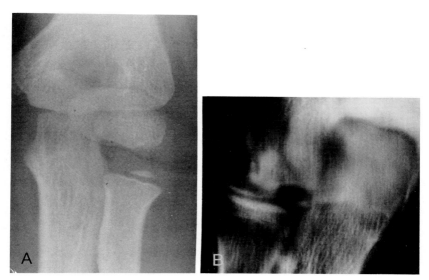

Figure 83. A. Radiograph of irregular capitellar ossification. B. Tomogram of defect in the lateral condyle of an adolescent with chronic elbow pain.

Elbow Dislocation

Figures 84–86

Anatomy
-Usually posterolateral

Clinical Diagnosis
-Swollen, often hyperextended

Radiologic Diagnosis
-Look for associated chondro-osseous damage (especially radial head or medial epicondyle)

Recommended Treatment
-Closed reduction
-May require open reduction/fixation of associated injuries

Complications
-Neurovascular damage
-Entrapment of medial epicondyle in joint
-Myositis ossificans
-Recurrent dislocation

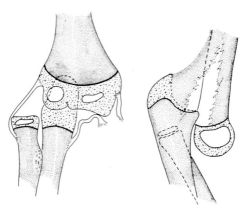

Figure 84. Schematic of elbow dislocation.

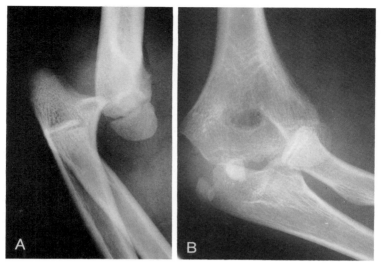

Figure 85. A. Posterior dislocation. B. Posterolateral dislocation with displacement of the avulsed medial epicondyle into the elbow joint.

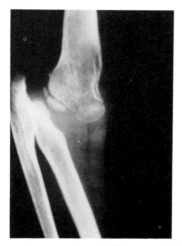

Figure 86. Appearance of an unreduced dislocated elbow two years after the initial injury.

References

Thompson HC, Garcia A: Myositis ossificans: aftermath of elbow injuries. Clin Orthop 50:129, 1967.

Wheeler, DK, Linscheid RL: Fracture-dislocations of the elbow. Clin Orthop 50:95, 1967.

Elbow
"Nursemaid's Elbow"

Anatomy
-Hyperpronation injury
-Ligamentous laxity
-Partial displacement of annular ligament

Clinical Diagnosis
-Child holds arm in pronation

Radiologic Diagnosis
-*Not* useful, other than to rule out other injuries (e.g., fracture of radial head)
-However, recent article (Frumkin) suggests a line drawn through the longitudinal axis of the radius may *not* bisect the capitellar ossification center

Recommended Treatment
-Gentle, but quick supination with your thumb on child's radial head

Complications
-Recurrence

References
Frumkin K: Nursemaid's elbow: a radiographic demonstration. Ann Emerg Med 14:690, 1985.
Salter R, Zaltz C: Anatomic investigations of the mechanism of injury and pathologic anatomy of "pulled elbow" in children. Clin Orthop 77:134, 1971.

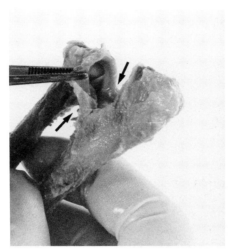

Figure 87. Anatomic specimen showing how annular ligament slips partially over the radial head to restrict forearm rotation, much like a torn meniscus may limit knee motion.

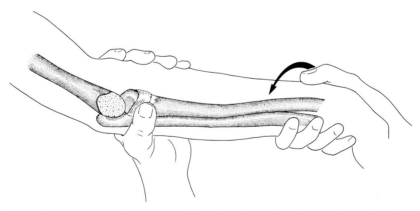

Figure 88. Method of reduction. The thumb is placed over the radial head and the forearm quickly supinated. This brings the partially displaced annular ligament back into its normal position around the radial neck.

Proximal Ulna Figure 89

Anatomy
-Late appearing secondary ossification center

Clinical Diagnosis
-Painful olecranon
-Inability to extend arm

Radiologic Diagnosis
-Look for separation of olecranon (metaphyseal fragment)
-Do not misinterpret a small secondary ossification center as a metaphyseal fracture fragment. Similarly, do not interpret a displaced metaphyseal fragment as a secondary ossification center

Treatment
-Usually open reduction, tension band fixation

Complications
-Refracture
-Non-union
-Disruption of "nontensile" fixation methods

Reference

Grantham SA, Kiernan HA: Displaced olecranon fracture in children. J Trauma 15:197, 1975.

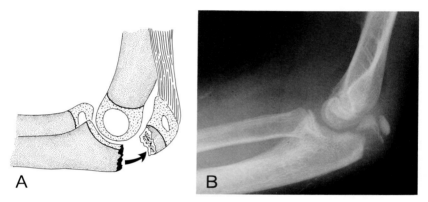

Figure 89. A. Schematic of proximal ulnar injury. B. Displaced proximal ulnar fracture.

Proximal Radius

Anatomy
-Susceptible intracapsular blood supply
-Metaphyseal compression injury most common pattern
-Physeal injuries are infrequent

Clinical Diagnosis
-Painful, swollen over radial head
-Loss of forearm rotation

Radiologic Diagnosis
-Assess degree of angular displacement

Treatment
-If metaphyseal, attempt closed manipulation with pressure over radial head
-Epiphyseal or physeal injuries usually require open reduction

Complications
-Metaphyseal: malunion may cause loss of supination/pronation
-Epiphyseal: avascular necrosis
-Epiphyseal: joint incongruency due to deformed radial head

Reference
Vahvanen V, Gripenberg L: Fracture of the radial neck in children. Acta Orthop Scand 49:32, 1978.

94   POCKET GUIDE TO PEDIATRIC FRACTURES

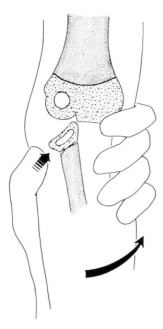

Figure 90. Schematic of proximal radial injury, showing placement of thumb during reduction.

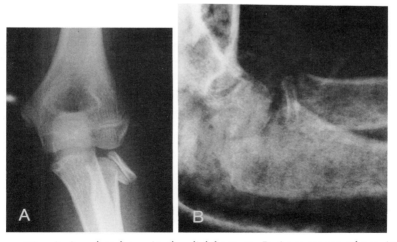

Figure 91. A. Angulated proximal radial fracture. B. Appearance of proximal radius following closed reduction.

Monteggia Injury

Anatomy
-Biomechanical interrelationships of radius and ulna "necessitate" some type of injury of both bones
-Usual pattern: radial head dislocation and proximal or middle third ulnar fracture

Clinical Diagnosis
-Radial head displacement not usually evident
-Pain over ulnar fracture

Radiologic Diagnosis
-Must obtain appropriate views of elbow to assess radio-humeral relationship when only an ulnar fracture (or even plastic bowing) occurs ANYWHERE along course of ulna
-May occur even when both bones are fractured

Treatment
-Adequate closed or open reduction of radial dislocation (ulna usually stable when radius reduced)

Complications
-Annular ligament disruption or displacement leading to unstable proximal radioulnar joint
-Incomplete reduction of radius
-FAILURE TO INITIALLY RECOGNIZE INJURY

Reference
Lloyd-Roberts GC, Bucknill TM: Anterior dislocation of the radial head in children. J Bone Joint Surg 59B:405, 1977.

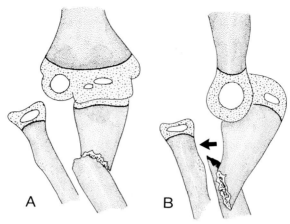

Figure 92. Schematics of a Monteggia injury, showing lateral displacement (A) and anterior displacement (B).

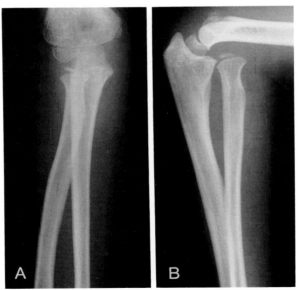

Figure 93. A. Deceptive appearance of this injury in the anteroposterior view. B. The lateral view readily demonstrates the radial head dislocation (unfortunately, 17 months after the ulnar fracture).

Radius and Ulna Diaphysis (Bowing)

Figures 94–95

Anatomy

-The changing microstructure of the radius and ulna make plastic deformation of one or both likely in the younger child

Clinical Diagnosis

-Pain in forearm

Radiologic Diagnosis

-Often difficult to assess since both bones may have normal curvature

Treatment

-Cast or splint for seven to ten days

Complications

-Unusual
-However, if not treated, the child may fall and convert it to a complete fracture

Reference

Crowe JE, Swischuk LE: Acute bowing fractures of the forearm in children: a frequently missed injury. Am J Roentgenol 128:981, 1977.

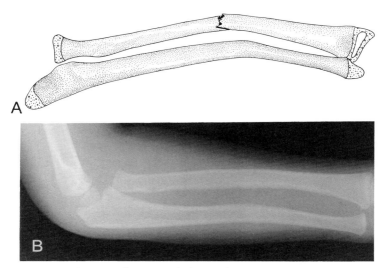

Figure 94. A. Schematic bowing of ulna with fracture of radius. B. Bowing of ulna with initially unrecognized dislocation of the radial head (Monteggia injury).

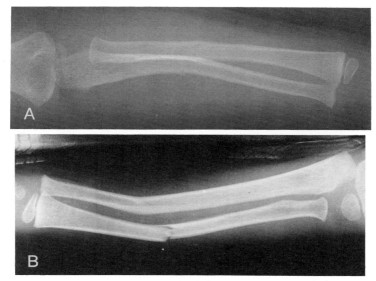

Figure 95. A. Bowing of both bones. B. Bowing of ulna.

Radius and Ulna Diaphysis (Greenstick)

Anatomy
-Typical pattern in young child with relatively porous diaphysis

Clinical Diagnosis
-Swelling, pain
-Sometimes deformity is palpable or visually evident

Radiologic Diagnosis
-Some of cortex intact

Treatment
-Three point pressure in cast necessary
-May require *completion* of fracture

Complications
-Angular change as swelling subsides and incomplete greenstick "springs" into an increasing deformity

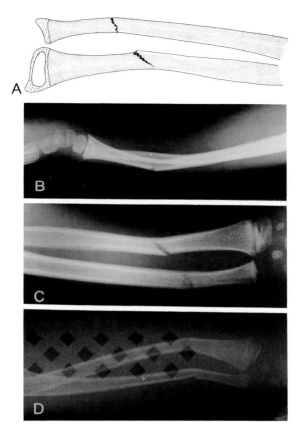

Figure 96. A. Schematic of greenstick fracture of the radius and complete fracture of the ulna. Note the plastic bowing of the intact cortex of the radius. B. Greenstick fracture of the radius. C. Greenstick fracture of one radial cortex, with separation of other cortex. D. Greenstick fracture of radius with a buckling (torus) type of greenstick fracture in the ulna.

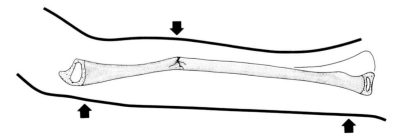

Figure 97. Three-point pressure in cast to counter the intact cortex.

Radius and Ulna Diaphysis (One Bone)

Anatomy
-Variable degree of cortical osteon bone in each allows different failure patterns
-Always assess at elbow (Monteggia injury) or wrist (Galeazzi injury) when only one bone is obviously fractured

Clinical Diagnosis
-Pain, swelling

Radiologic Diagnosis
-Get oblique views to rule out small, undisplaced greenstick fracture or bowing of other bone
-Beware of wrist, elbow injuries

Treatment
-Use intact bone as internal splint
-Closed reduction usually possible

Complications
-Unusual
-Missing associated proximal or distal injury

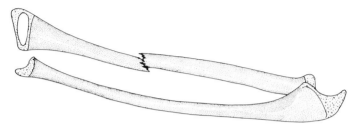

Figure 98. Schematic of fracture of the radius associated with an intact ulna.

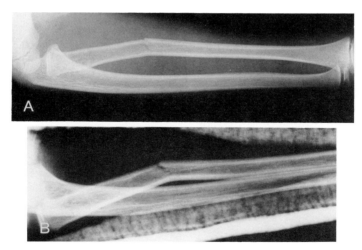

Figure 99. A. Greenstick fracture of the radius with an intact ulna. B. "Reduced" greenstick radial fracture with intact ulna. This degree of angulation is unacceptable as it may restrict forearm rotation.

Radius and Ulna Diaphysis (Both Bones)

Figures 100–102

Anatomy
-Fracture patterns change as the cortex matures
-Greenstick pattern more common prior to ten years of age
-Complete fracture more common after ten years of age

Clinical Diagnosis
-Angular deformity common

Radiologic Diagnosis
-Assess fracture patterns, degree of displacement, and any overriding

Treatment
-Closed reduction under ten years
-Open reduction, internal fixation more likely in child older than ten years

Complications
-Malunion
-Non-union of one or both bones
-Decreased pronation/supination

Reference
Darawulla J: A study of radioulnar movements following fractures of the forearm in children. Clin Orthop 139:114, 1979.

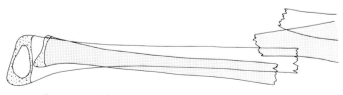

Figure 100. Schematic of fracture of both bones of the forearm, with displacement and overriding.

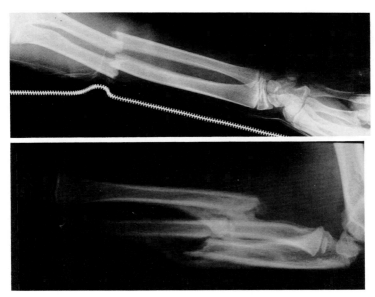

Figure 101. Top. Fracture of both bones. Bottom. Callus formation in patient with fractures of radius and ulna.

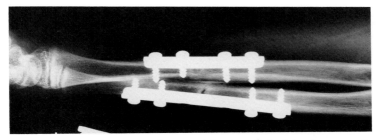

Figure 102. Open reduction and internal fixation (ORIF) for fracture of radius and ulna in teenager.

Radius and Ulna Distal Metaphysis

Anatomy
-One of most frequently injured areas
-Torus injury common
-Periosteum intact dorsally, disrupted on volar surface
-Bone may herniate into or through pronator quadratus

Clinical Diagnosis
-"Silver spoon" deformity when displaced
-Painful, variably swollen wrist
-Assess median nerve carefully

Radiologic Diagnosis
-Evaluate extent of fracture (torus to dorsally displaced)

Treatment
-Torus: splint for approximately two weeks
-Angulated: correct deformity
-Dorsally displaced: closed reduction by "walking" the distal fragment
-Reassess after a few days to be certain angulation does not recur

Complications
-Failure to reduce displacement (may require open reduction)
-Look at ulnar styloid (may develop non-union)
-Angulation

Reference
Levinthal DH: Fractures of the lower one third of both bones of the forearm in children. Surg Gynec Obstet 57:790, 1933.

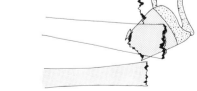

Figure 103.   Schematic of dorsally displaced distal metaphyseal fractures.

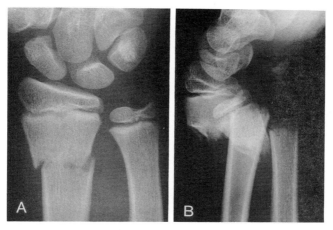

Figure 104. A. Radiograph of distal metaphyseal fracture. B. Displaced distal metaphyseal fracture.

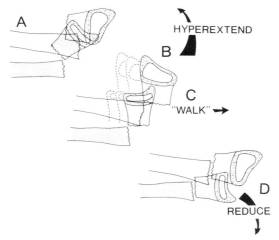

Figure 105. Schematic of hyperextension method of reduction of the dorsally displaced, overriding distal metaphyseal fracture.

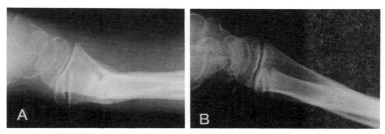

Figure 106. A. Recurrent angulation which occurred when patient did not return for scheduled follow-up until four weeks had elapsed following injury. B. Remodeling in the same patient three years later has corrected the malunion.

Radius
Distal Physis

Anatomy
-One of most common physeal injuries
-Usually type 1 or 2 pattern

Clinical Diagnosis
-Pain, swelling over distal radius

Radiologic Diagnosis
-Variably displaced
-May require oblique views to see metaphyseal fragment
-Look at ulnar styloid

Treatment
-GENTLE closed reduction

Complications
-Growth slowdown or arrest
-Ulnar styloid non-union (delayed appearance; rarely painful)

Reference
Bradgon RA: Fractures of the distal radial epiphysis. Clin Orthop 41:59, 1965.

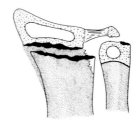

Figure 107.   Schematic of distal physeal fracture associated with ulnar styloid fracture.

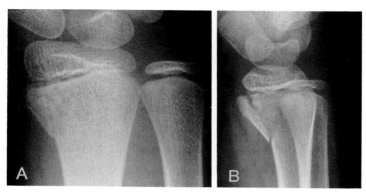

Figure 108. Anteroposterior (A) and oblique (B) views of minimally displaced physeal injury.

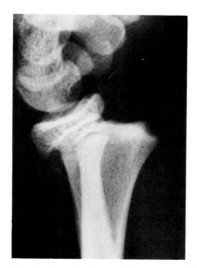

Figure 109. Moderately displaced physeal fracture. Relaxation should be used before reduction to minimize physeal damage during manipulation.

Ulna
Distal Physis

Anatomy
-Susceptible vascular supply

Clinical Diagnosis
-Infrequent injury

Radiologic Diagnosis
-Assess degree of displacement

Treatment
-Closed reduction
-When completely displaced usually requires open reduction

Complications
-Growth arrest leading to short ulna
-May adversely affect development of distal radius

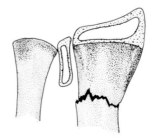

Figure 110.   Schematic of displaced distal ulnar physeal injury.

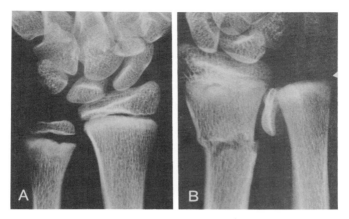

Figure 111. A. Separated, but undisplaced type 1 ulnar physeal injury. B. Displaced physeal injury.

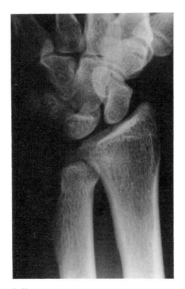

Figure 112. Deformity following complete growth arrest after distal ulnar fracture.

Wrist
Carpal Navicular

Anatomy
-Surrounding cartilage decreases susceptibility to fracture
-Avulsion injuries most common, especially in adolescent

Clinical Diagnosis
-Pain in anatomic "snuffbox"

Radiologic Diagnosis
-Take sufficient views
-Follow-up films necessary to rule out fracture at chondro-osseous junction

Recommended Treatment
-Thumb spica cast if painful in snuffbox (even if radiograph is "normal")

Complications
-Ischemic necrosis rare (more likely in teenager)

References

Larson B., Light TR, Ogden JA: Fracture and ischemic necrosis of the immature scaphoid. J Hand Surg 12A:122, 1987.

Mussbichler H: Injuries of the carpal scaphoid in children. Acta Radiol (Diagn) 56:361, 1961.

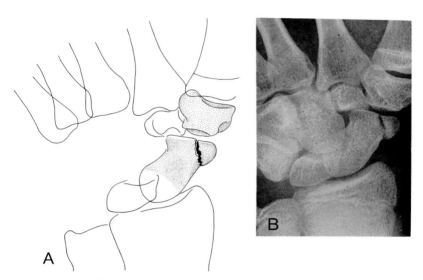

Figure 113. A. Schematic of navicular fracture. B. Typical adolescent fracture of the navicula.

Thumb Dislocation

Anatomy
-Much less capsular and ligamentous injury compared to adult
-Entrapment by tendons around neck of metacarpal

Clinical Diagnosis
-Fixed hyperextension deformity usually obvious

Radiologic Diagnosis
-Accompanying fracture unlikely

Recommended Treatment
-Closed reduction
-Open reduction rarely necessary

Complications
-Chronic instability

Reference
Green DP: Hand injuries in children. Pediatr Clin North Am 24:903, 1977.

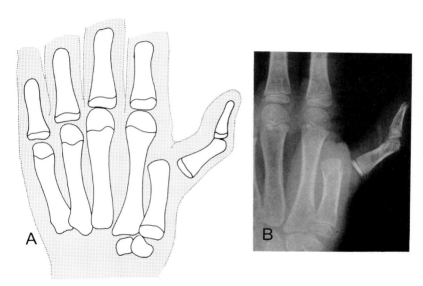

Figure 114. A. Schematic. B. Radiograph of thumb metacarpophalangeal dislocation.

Thumb
Bennett's Fracture

Anatomy
-Type 2 injury with a metaphyseal fragment creates the analogue of the
 adult injury

Clinical Diagnosis
-Painful swelling at base of thumb

Radiologic Diagnosis
-Assess size of metaphyseal fracture
-Assess degree of displacement

Recommended Treatment
-Closed reduction with or without percutaneous pinning
-Open reduction may be frequently necessary

Complications
-Angulation (malunion)
-Delayed union

Reference
Griffiths JC: Bennett's fracture in childhood. Br J Clin Pract 20:582, 1967.

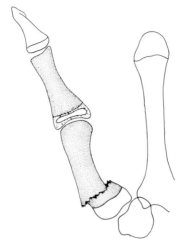

Figure 115. Schematic of childhood Bennett's fracture.

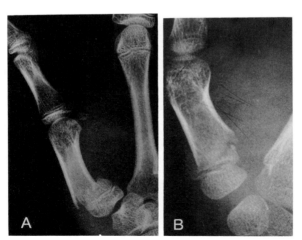

Figure 116. A. Radiograph of metaphyseal pattern. B. Radiograph of physeal pattern.

Hand
Metacarpal Fracture
(Diaphysis)

Figure 117

Anatomy
-Either transverse or spiral, usually with minimal displacement

Clinical Diagnosis
-Painful swelling, especially over dorsum of hand

Radiologic Diagnosis
-May require oblique views, especially if fracture is incomplete

Recommended Treatment
-Closed reduction
-Well padded splint
-Elevation
-May require pin fixation if angulation is significant

Complications
-Infection

Reference
Wood VE: Fractures of the hand in children. Orthop Clin North Am 7:527, 1976.

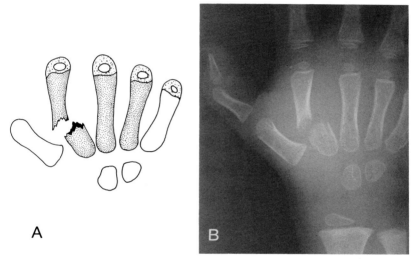

A

B

Figure 117. A. Schematic of metacarpal fracture. B. Radiograph of fracture of diaphysis of the second metacarpal.

Hand
Metacarpal Fracture
(Distal)

Anatomy
-Unusual injuries in digits 2 to 4
-Common as "boxer's" fracture in digit 5 (little finger)

Clinical Diagnosis
-Loss of knuckle prominence

Radiologic Diagnosis
-Usually volar displacement with metaphyseal crushing or physeal displacement

Recommended Treatment
-Closed reduction of angular displacement
-Open reduction if physis or epiphysis injured

Complications
-Failure to correct angulation
-Avascular necrosis
-Growth slowdown or arrest leading to short metacarpal

Reference
Light TR, Ogden JA: Metacarpal epiphyseal fractures. J Hand Surg, in press.

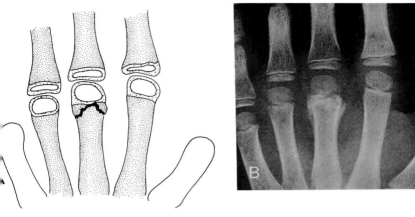

Figure 118. A. Schematic. B. Radiograph of physeal injury of the index metacarpal.

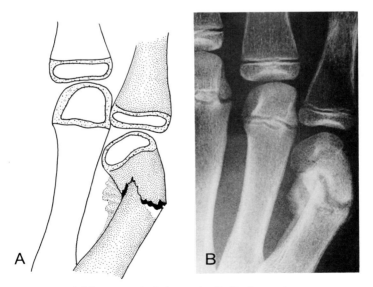

Figure 119. "Boxer's" fracture. A. Schematic. B. Radiograph.

Hand Metacarpophalangeal Dislocation

Figure 120

Anatomy
-Involves index or little finger

Clinical Diagnosis
-Prominent metacarpal head in palmar space

Radiologic Diagnosis
-Best viewed in lateral or oblique

Recommended Treatment
-Open reduction
-Treat quickly to avoid potential vascular compromise

Complications
-Failure to recognize
-Failure to reduce
-Ischemic necrosis

Reference

Green DP, Terry GC: Complex dislocation of the metacarpophalangeal joint—correlative pathological anatomy. J Bone Joint Surg 55A:1480, 1973.

Light TR, Ogden JA: Complex dislocation of the index metacarpophalangeal joint in the skeletally immature patient. J Hand Surg, in press.

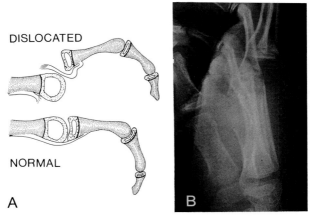

Figure 120. A. Schematic. B. Metacarpophalangeal dislocation of index finger in a ten-year-old.

Hand
Phalangeal Physis

Anatomy
-Involves proximal ends of phalanges
-Type of injuries represent chondro-osseous failure of the collateral
 ligament insertions. Actual interligamentous disruption is unusual

Clinical Diagnosis
-Similar appearance to interphalangeal dislocation

Radiologic Diagnosis
-Assess fracture pattern and extent of displacement

Recommended Treatment
-Closed reduction, types 1, 2
-Open reduction if articular surface is involved (types 3, 4, 7)

Complications
-Joint disruption
-Growth damage with shortening or angulation
-Collateral instability

Reference
Bora FW Jr, Nissenbaum M, Ignatius P: The treatment of epiphyseal fracture of the hand.
  Orthop Digest 5:11, 1976.

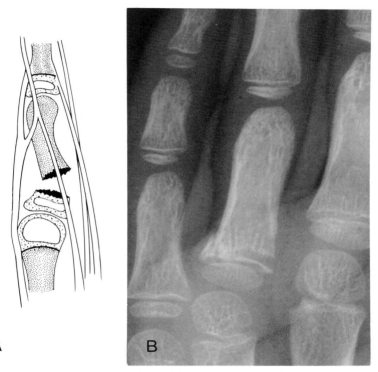

Figure 121. A. Schematic. B. Physeal fracture (type 2) of the proximal phalanx.

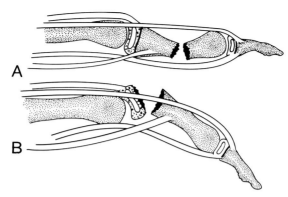

Figure 122. Schematics of shaft (A) and physeal (B) fractures involving the middle phalanx.

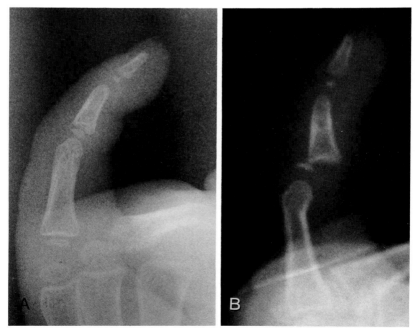

Figure 123. A. Undisplaced injury of the middle phalangeal physis. B. Displacement is evident; the patient removed the splint the day following injury and returned to clinic three weeks later. The displacement was irreducible.

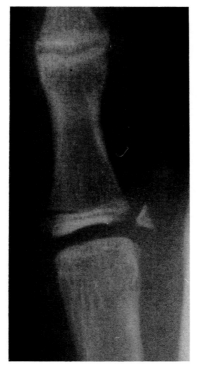

Figure 124. Type 7 injury. This is the typical pattern of collateral ligament failure as a chondro-osseous, rather than ligamentous, injury.

Hand
Extra-Octave Fracture

Anatomy
-Involvement of proximal phalanx, little finger

Clinical Diagnosis
-Ulnar deviation of little finger

Radiologic Diagnosis
-Usually a physeal fracture (may be type 1 or 2)

Recommended Treatment
-Closed reduction with pencil between fourth and fifth digits
-Alternatively, flex metacarpophalangeal joint to 90 degrees and radially
 displace the digit

Complications
-Persistent ulnar angulation
-Growth injury (rare)

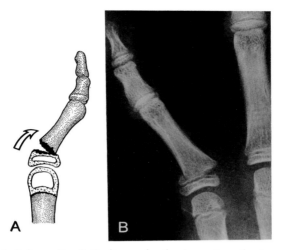

Figure 125. A. Schematic. B. Radiograph of extra-octave fracture.

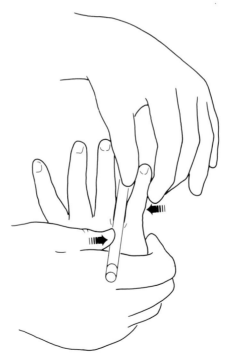

Figure 126. Method of reduction (web space).

Hand Interphalangeal Dislocation

Figure 127

Anatomy
-Ligamentous laxity allows displacement without significant soft tissue injury

Clinical Diagnosis
-"Step-like" joint without motion

Radiologic Diagnosis
-Dislocation evident
-Look for peripheral avulsions of small segments of secondary ossification centers

Recommended Treatment
-Closed reduction
-Open fixation if a significant osseous fragment evident

Complications
-Joint instability (usually on lateral sides)
-Entrapment of volar plate
-Recurrent dislocation

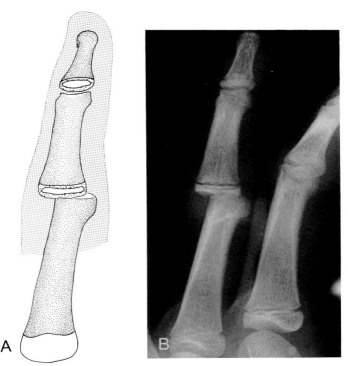

Figure 127. A. Schematic of interphalangeal dislocation. B. Radiograph.

Hand
Phalanx (Condyle)

Anatomy
-Tendency to rotate up to 90 degrees due to ligaments

Clinical Diagnosis
-Pain, swelling at joint (distal end of phalanx)

Radiologic Diagnosis
-Anteroposterior may appear to be normal
-Lateral is essential—to assess extent of rotational disruption

Treatment
-Closed, if undisplaced, with frequent follow-up
-Percutaneous fixation if relatively unstable
-Open reduction with significant rotation

Complications
-Delayed or non-union
-Malunion

Reference

Dixon GL, Moon NF: Rotational supracondylar fractures of the proximal phalanx in children. Clin Orthop 83:151, 1972.

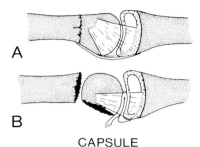

CAPSULE

Figure 128. Schematic of undisplaced (A) and rotationally displaced (B) condylar fractures.

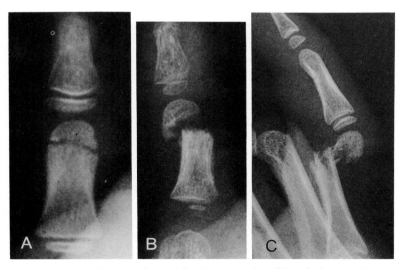

Figure 129. A. Undisplaced condylar fracture of middle phalanx. B,C. Anteroposterior and lateral views of displaced condylar fracture.

Hand
Mallet Finger

Figures 130–132

Anatomy
-Avulsion of extensor mechanism
-Usually includes part or all of epiphysis, in contrast to adults with pure soft tissue injury
-Pattern of fracture relates to extent of skeletal maturation

Clinical Diagnosis
-Inability to spontaneously extend the distal end of the finger, with or without resistance

Radiologic Diagnosis
-Type 1 injury in young child
-Type 3 injury in adolescent

Recommended Treatment
-Closed reduction with hyperextension splint. However, take an x-ray to be certain reduction is complete (see Fig. 132B)
-Open reduction if type 1 (entire epiphysis) cannot be satisfactorily reduced
-Open reduction and internal fixation (ORIF) if physeal or joint involvement is significant (e.g., type 3 injury)

Complications
-Growth arrest
-Failure to reduce fragment
-Inability to hyperextend
-Excessive bone

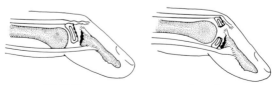

CHILD   ADOLESCENT

Figure 130.   Schematic of childhood and adolescent variations.

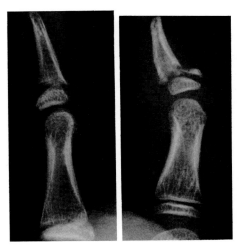

Figure 131. Type 1 (left) and type 2 (right) growth plate patterns in children.

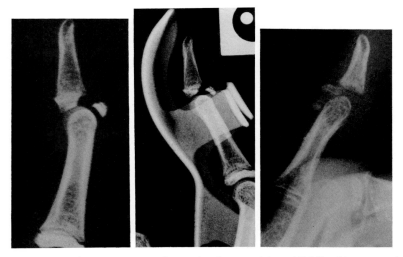

Figure 132. Left. Type 3 growth mechanism avulsion. Middle. Unacceptable reduction in "cock-up" splint. Right. Chronic non-union.

Hand
Distal Phalanx (Tuft)

Figure 133

Anatomy
-Disruption of pulp space and septae

Clinical Diagnosis
-Often an open injury
-Accompanying nail injury

Radiologic Diagnosis
-Comminution is common

Recommended Treatment
-Splint
-Soft tissue care
-Antibiotics

Complications
-Osteomyelitis
-Nail damage

References
Enger WD, Glancy WG: Traumatic avulsion of the fingernail associated with injury to the phalangeal epiphyseal plate. J Bone Joint Surg 60A:713, 1978.
Samdzem SC: Management of the acute fingertip injury in the child. Hand 6:190, 1974.

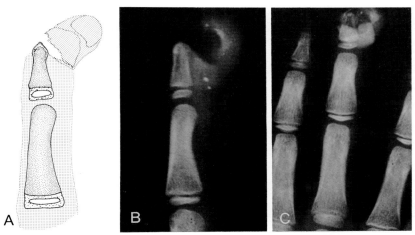

Figure 133. A. Schematic of open tuft injury. B. Radiologic appearance. C. Ectopic bone formation three weeks after injury.

Spine
C1

Figure 134

Anatomy
-Develops three cartilaginous junctions (synchondroses)
-These synchondroses disappear by four to five years
-The anterior ossification center appears postnatally during the first year of life

Clinical Diagnosis
-Evaluate the upper cervical spine carefully whenever there is head injury or neck pain

Radiologic Diagnosis
-Fracture of the ring
-Cross sectional imaging best (CT, MRI)

Recommended Treatment
-Requires adequate immobilization
-In an active child a *minerva jacket is most effective* (the fracture usually heals within six to eight weeks)

Complications
-High level brain stem injury
-Non-union unlikely
-Recurrent instability unlikely

Reference
Ogden JA: Radiology of postnatal skeletal development. XI. The first cervical vertebra. Skel Radiol 12:169, 1984.

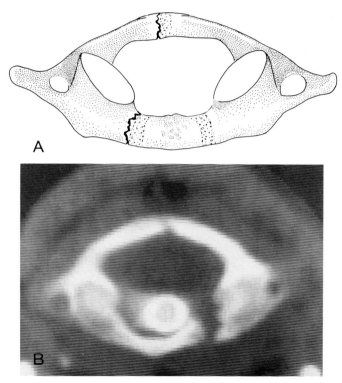

Figure 134. A. Schematic of anterior and posterior arch fractures of C1. B. Radiography (CT) of injury in a six-year-old.

Spine
C1/C2 Rotational Subluxation

Figures 135–136

Anatomy
-Normal ligamentous laxity allows considerable displacement in rotation
-Muscle spasm probably a significant factor in "locking" the displacement

Clinical Diagnosis
-Torticollis

Radiologic Diagnosis
-Usually evident by different views of head versus lower cervical spine
-Cross sectional imaging excellent
-Concomitant fracture unlikely

Recommended Treatment
-Traction
-Gentle manipulation (without anesthesia)
-Acute or even chronic delayed diagnosis of rotatory subluxation must be treated first by gentle traction (i.e., head halter), and only if unsuccessful by manipulative reduction

Complications
-Fixed subluxation
-Spinal cord or brain stem injury

References

Fielding JW, Cochran GVB, Lawsing JF, Hohl M: Tears of the transverse ligament of the atlas: a clinical and biomechanical study. J Bone Joint Surg 56A:1683–1691, 1974.

Ogden JA, Murphy MJ, Southwick WO, Ogden DA: Radiology of postnatal skeletal development. XIII. C1/C2 interrelationships. Skel Radiol 15:433, 1986.

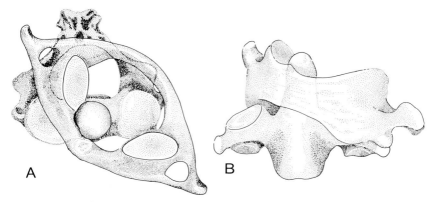

Figure 135. Schematics of rotational displacement from above (A) and frontal (B) projections.

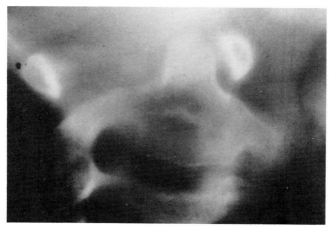

Figure 136. Tomography of a rotational displacement.

Spine
C2

Anatomy
-Paired posterior and single anterior center
-Separate dens ossification
-Dentocentral synchondrosis
-Ossiculum terminale appears during adolescence

Clinical Diagnosis
-Restricted neck motion
-Torticollis

Radiologic Diagnosis
-Fracture at level of growth plate
-Must distinguish fracture from dentocentral synchondrosis

Recommended Treatment
-Immobilization (e.g., Minerva jacket)

Complications
-Development of os odontoideum
-Spinal cord injury

References

Griffiths SC: Fracture of the odontoid process in children. J Pediatr Surg 7:680–683, 1972.
Ogden JA: Radiology of postnatal skeletal development. XII. The second cervical vertebra. Skel Radiol 12:169, 1984.
Sherk HH, Nicholson JT: Fractures of the odontoid process in young children. J Bone Joint Surg 60A:921–924, 1978.

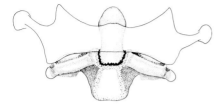

Figure 137. Schematic of fracture following course of physis between the dens and body of C2.

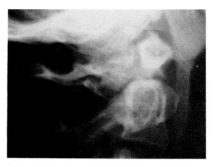

Figure 139. Os odontoideum noted two years after an "innocuous" neck injury and "negative" cervical spine.

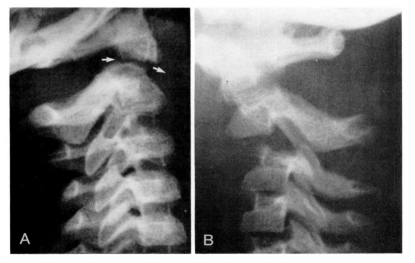

Figure 138. A. Fracture of dens with anterior displacement (arrows) of the dens. B. Similar case, with rapid healing in six weeks.

Spine
Lower Cervical

Anatomy
-Changing angulation of facet joints
-Changing interspinous ligamentous laxity
-"Ring" apophysis

Clinical Diagnosis
-Restricted neck motion
-Pain

Radiologic Diagnosis
-Hypermobility may cause pseudosubluxation
-Anterior sloping of superior margin must not be confused with compression fracture
-Anterior displacement of ossification ("ring apophysis")

Recommended Treatment
-Collar or cast
-Anterior fusions generally contraindicated
-Limited posterior interspinous fusion when necessary

Complications
-Growth arrest causing angular deformation
-Neural damage (spinal cord or roots)

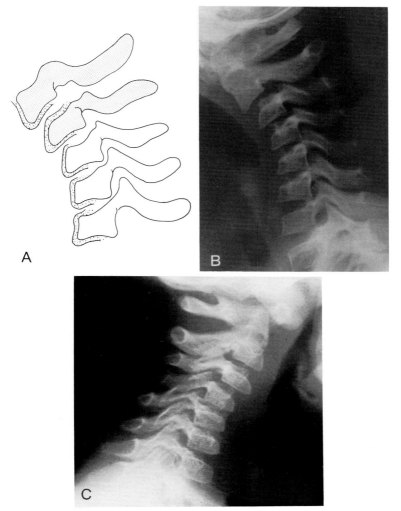

Figure 140. Hypermobility. A. Schematic. B,C. Variations of mobility in normal children.

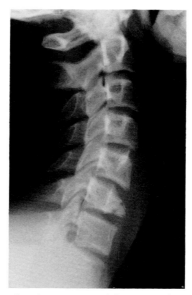

Figure 141. Anterior wedge (compression) fracture of C6.

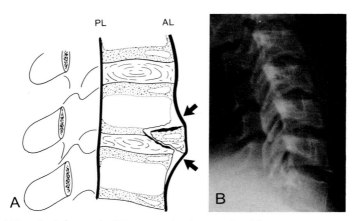

Figure 142. A. Schematic (AL—anterior longitudinal ligament; PL—posterior longitudinal ligament). B. Radiograph of anterior avulsion of the ring "apophysis" of C7 following a hyperextension injury.

References

Bailey DK: The normal cervical spine in infants and children. Radiology 59:712–719, 1952.

Cattell HS, Filtzer DS: Pseudosubluxation and other normal variations in the cervical spine in children. J Bone Joint Surg 47A:1295–1309, 1965.

Lawson JP, Ogden JA, Bucholz RW: Physeal injuries of the cervical spine. J. Pediatr Orthop, in press.

Sherk HH, Schut L: Fractures and dislocations of the cervical spine in children. Orthop Clin North Am 7:593–604, 1976.

Sullivan CR, Bruwer AJ, Harris LE: Hypermobility of the cervical spine in children: a pitfall in the diagnosis of cervical dislocation. Am J Surg 95:636–640, 1958.

Spine
Thoracolumbar

Anatomy
-Hypermobility may allow facet displacement
-Ability of vertebral body to restore some or all of height if compressed
 anteriorly

Clinical Diagnosis
-Back pain
-Neurologic deficit

Radiologic Diagnosis
-Some injuries subtle (may spontaneously reduce)
-Anteroposterior/lateral view will visualize basic injury
-Use cross sectional techniques to assess canal impingement, narrowing

Recommended Treatment
-Stabilization of fracture or facet disruption
-Often requires surgical intervention

Complications
-Spinal cord or root injury

References

Hachen HJ: Spinal cord injury in children and adolescents. Diagnostic pitfalls and
    therapeutic considerations in the acute stage. Paraplegia 15:55–64, 1977–78.
Kewalramani LS, Tori JA: Spinal cord trauma in children: neurological patterns, radiologic
    features and pathomechanics of injury. Spine 5:11–18, 1980.
Walsh JW, Stevens DB, Young AB: Traumatic paraplegia in children without contiguous
    spinal fracture or dislocation. Neurosurgery 12:439–445, 1983.

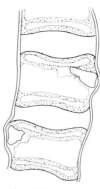

Figure 143. Schematic of typical crush injuries involving vertebral body "corners" in child.

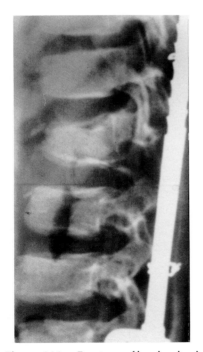

Figure 144. Fracture of lumbar body treated by rod fixation/ stabilization.

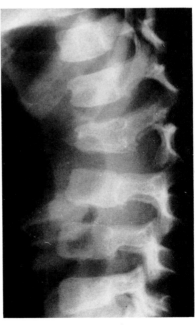

Figure 145. Facet disruption and posterior element fracture at the thoracolumbar junction.

Spine
Lumbar Apophysis

Anatomy
-Posterior apophysis and secondary ossification center develop during adolescence

Clinical Diagnosis
-Back pain, often mimicking sciatica
-Herniated disc an infrequent injury
-Often seen in teenage weight lifters

Radiologic Diagnosis
-Posteriorly displaced fragment of bone, usually from inferior margin
-Use cross-sectional imaging to assess canal impingement

Recommended Treatment
-Usually requires removal of fragment

Complications
-Failure to make the diagnosis
-Permanent narrowing of canal (spinal stenosis)

Reference

Handel SF, Twiford TW Jr, Reigel DH, Kaufman KH: Posterior lumbar apophyseal fractures. Radiology 130:629–633, 1979.

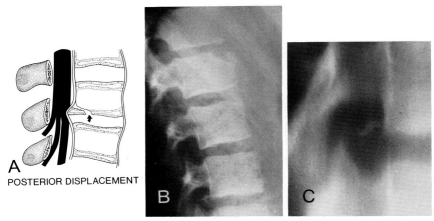

POSTERIOR DISPLACEMENT

Figure 146. A. Schematic. B. Displaced fragment at L4-5. Note the anterior Scheuermann's lesion involving L2. C. Magnification view showing small fragment in the canal.

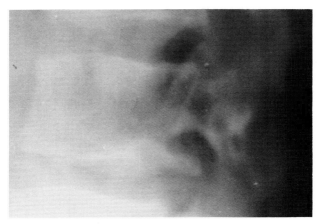

Figure 147. Osseous healing of avulsed fragment. This led to chronic sciatic symptoms.

Pelvis
Rami

Anatomy
-Rami should be considered analogous to a long bone with an epiphysis at either end
-Evaluate sacroiliac region (dislocation versus chondro-osseous separation), as entire hemipelvis may be involved
-Displacement of rami should be considered a growth mechanism injury
-Periosteal sleeve may be intact and eventually will fill in the apparent radiologic defect

Clinical Diagnosis
-Assess possible visceral injury (bladder, urethra)

Radiologic Diagnosis
-CT scan important to assess posterior displacement
-Apparent widening of symphysis pubis is usually a physeal separation

Recommended Treatment
-Complete evaluation for internal injury (especially bladder, urethra)
-Bed rest
-Progressive weight bearing (fractures heal rapidly)
-External fixation may be necessary
-Embolization for excessive hemorrhage

Complications
-Visceral damage
-Urethral damage: greater incidence in males
-Vascular:extensive blood loss

References

Barlow B, Rottenberg RW, Santulli TV: Angiographic diagnosis and treatment of bleeding by selective embolization following pelvic fractures in children. J Pediatr Surg 10:939, 1975.

Quinby, WC: Fractures of the pelvis and other associated injuries in children. J Pediatr Surg 1:353, 1966.

Watts H: Fractures of the pelvis in children. Orthop Clin North Am 7:615, 1976.

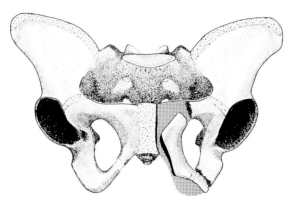

Figure 148. Schematic of rami avulsion with relatively intact periosteal sleeve.

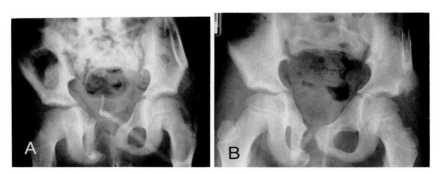

Figure 149. Avulsion of rami (A) with "filling-in" of apparent diastasis several weeks later (B).

Pelvis
Acetabulum (Triradiate Cartilage)

Anatomy
-Three "armed" cartilage within the acetabulum

Clinical Diagnosis
-Restricted hip range of motion
-May require column (Judet) views

Radiologic Diagnosis
-Difficult to observe radiographically

Recommended Treatment
-Bed rest, followed by four to six weeks of nonweight bearing
-Serial roentgenographic follow-up
-Infrequently requires open reduction

Complications
-Premature closure of triradiate cartilage leading to shallow acetabulum
 and subluxation of femoral head
-May require reconstruction (e.g., osteotomy, shelf)

Reference
Bucholz RW, Ezaki M, Ogden JA: Injury to the acetabular triradiate physeal cartilage. J
  Bone Joint Surg 64-A:600–609, 1982.

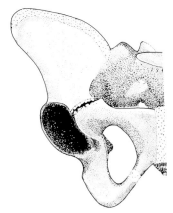

Figure 150. Schematic of triradiate injury.

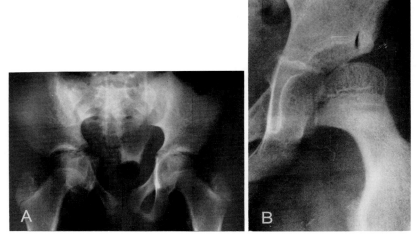

Figure 151. A. Fracture-separation of triradiate in an adolescent. B. Premature epiphyseodesis complicating triradiate injury.

Pelvis
Iliac Spines

Figure 152

Anatomy
-Traction "apophysis" at origin of major thigh and leg musculature

Clinical Diagnosis
-Often termed "hip pointer" by coach or trainer
-Usually occurs during athletic activity

Radiologic Diagnosis
-Displacement of osseous fragment: may be either secondary, ossification center or metaphyseal bone
-Impossible to diagnose if only the cartilaginous portion is avulsed; however, the subsequent callus makes the fracture evident

Recommended Treatment
-Discontinue sports activity
-Crutches with progressive weight bearing for three to six weeks
-Reconditioning for musculature involved in the particular sporting activity

Complications
-Exostosis
-Chronic pain

Reference
Godshall RW, Hansen CA: Incomplete avulsion of a portion of the iliac epiphysis. An injury of young athletes. J Bone Joint Surg 55-A:1301, 1973.

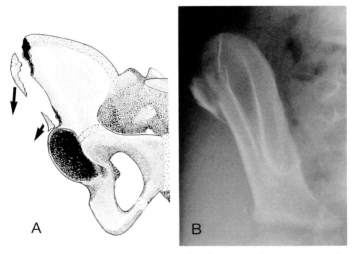

Figure 152. A. Schematic of superior and inferior avulsions. B. Avulsion of superior iliac spine.

Pelvis
Ischium

Figure 153

Anatomy
-Major origin of hamstrings
-"Apophyseal" injury

Clinical Diagnosis
-Pain over tuberosity, following either chronic exertion or acute injury

Radiologic Diagnosis
-May have irregular bone formation if a chronic injury
-Must distinguish from tumor or osteomyelitis

Recommended Treatment
-Discontinuation of sports until asymptomatic
-Significant displacement may require surgical fixation

Complications
-Non-union of fragment (with pain)
-Sciatic nerve injury (may be from chronic impingement)

References

Martin TA, Pipkin E: Treatment of avulsion of the ischial tuberosity. Clin Orthop 10:108–118, 1957.
Milch H: Ischial apophysiolysis. Clin Orthop 2:184–193, 1953.

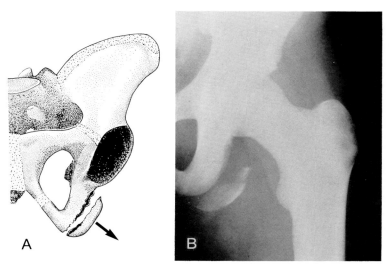

Figure 153. A. Schematic of ischial avulsion. B. Avulsion and displacement of ischial tuberosity.

Hip
Dislocation

Figures 154–156

Anatomy

-Relatively stable ball-and-socket joint
-Normal laxity in child may contribute to dislocation with minimal, if any, trauma
-Dislocation usually posterior; anterior much less common

Clinical Diagnosis

-Shortened, adducted leg (posterior dislocation)
-Shortened, abducted leg (anterior dislocation)

Radiologic Diagnosis

-Displacement of femoral head
-Look for peripheral acetabular fracture (posteriorly), but do NOT confuse with normal secondary ossification centers appearing during adolescence

Recommended Treatment

-Closed reduction
-Open reduction when necessary
-Nonweight bearing for three to four weeks

Complications

-Rim cartilage disruption preventing anatomic reduction
-Recurrent dislocation
-Ischemic necrosis
-Acute slipped capital femoral epiphysis during reduction

References

Barquet A: A natural history of avascular necrosis following traumatic hip dislocation in childhood. Acta Orthop Scand 53:815–820, 1982.

Ofierski CM: Traumatic dislocation of the hip in children. J Bone Joint Surg 63B:194–197, 1981.

Pennsylvania Orthopaedic Society: Traumatic dislocation of the hip in children. J Bone Joint Surg 50A:79–89, 1968.

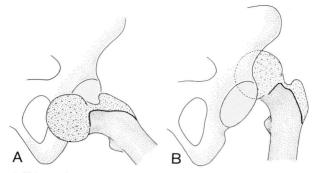

Figure 154. Schematics of anterior (A) and posterior (B) hip dislocation.

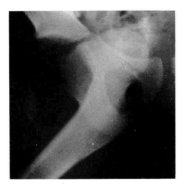

Figure 155. Radiograph of anterior dislocation.

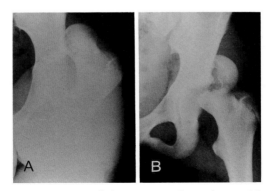

Figure l56. A. Posterosuperior dislocation. B. Slipped capital femoral epiphysis following attempted reduction.

Femur
Proximal Physis

Figures 157–159

Anatomy

-Capital femur and greater trochanter have variable cartilaginous continuity, causing differing morphologic lesions
-In the neonate both regions are injured together, whereas the older child only sustains injury to the capital femoral physis

Clinical Diagnosis

-Painful hip motion

Radiologic Diagnosis

-May only have slight widening of the capital femoral physis
-In neonate, confusion with congenital dysplasia of the hip

Recommended Treatment

-Aspiration of hip joint
-May require capsulotomy to decrease pressure
-Closed reduction in infant
-Older child may require internal fixation (use smooth pins to allow for growth)

Complications

-Ischemic necrosis
-Premature closure of physis

References

Ogden JA, Lee KE, Rudicel SA, Pelker RR: Proximal femoral epiphysiolysis in the neonate. J Ped Orthop 4:285–292, 1984.
Ratliff AHC: Traumatic separation of the upper femoral epiphysis in young children. J Bone Joint Surg 55B:757–770, 1968.

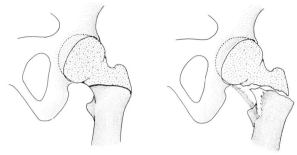

Figure 157. Schematic of neonatal injury.

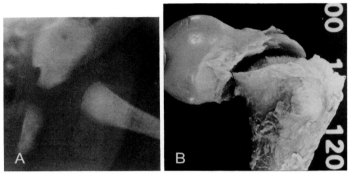

Figure 158. A. Neonatal injury, which appears to be a dislocation. However, the acetabular index is normal. B. Specimen showing how the entire proximal femoral epiphysis is displaced.

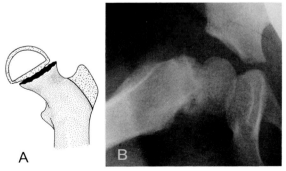

Figure 159. A. Schematic of physeal injury in older child. B. Physeal fracture in a four-year-old (seven weeks after the injury).

Femur
Slipped Capital Femoral Epiphysis

Figures 160–161

Anatomy
-Usually a chronic injury in the adolescent
-May occur acutely following a fall, heavy contact in athletics
-Infrequently may occur during attempted reduction of hip dislocation

Clinical Diagnosis
-Beware when there is pain anywhere between groin and knee

Radiologic Diagnosis
-Lateral is the most diagnostic view; anteroposterior may appear normal
-Bone scan

Recommended Treatment
-Traction for relief of joint irritation and gradual spontaneous reduction
-Possible *gentle* manipulative reduction of acute injury
-Internal fixation

Complications
-Ischemic necrosis
-Cartilage necrosis (chondrolysis)
-Joint deformity

Reference
Fahey JJ, O'Brien ET: Acute slipped capital femoral epiphysis. J Bone Joint Surg 47A:1105, 1965.

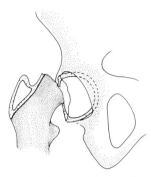

Figure 160. Schematic of slipped capital femoral epiphysis.

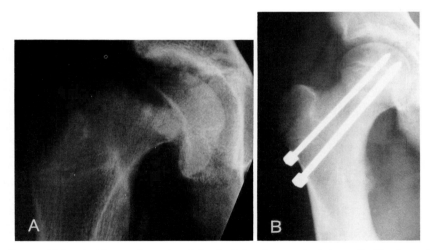

Figure 161. A. Varus slipped epiphysis following acute injury. B. Pinning of acute slipped capital femoral epiphysis.

Femur
Femoral Neck

Figures 162–164

Anatomy
-Injury to neck cartilage
-Injury to vessels supplying femoral head

Clinical Diagnosis
-Painful hip motion
-Leg is externally rotated when fracture is complete

Radiologic Diagnosis
-Assess degree of displacement

Recommended Treatment
-Traction
-Internal fixation
-Possible capsulotomy (for needle aspiration)

Complications
-Non-union
-Delayed union
-Coxa vara
-Ischemic necrosis

References

Canale ST, Bourland WL: Fracture of the neck and intertrochanteric region of the femur in children. J Bone Joint Surg 59A:431–443, 1977.

Lam SF: Fractures of the neck of the femur in children. J Bone Joint Surg 53A:1165–1179, 1971.

Ratliff AHC: Fractures of the neck of the femur in children. In: The Hip, Proceedings of the Ninth Open Scientific Meeting of the Hip Society. CV Mosby, St. Louis, 1981.

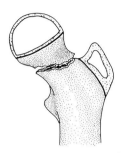

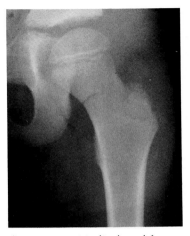

Figure 162. Schematic of femoral neck fracture.

Figure 163. Undisplaced fracture.

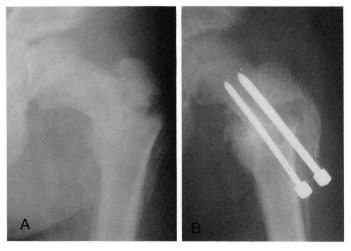

Figure 164. A. Displaced femoral neck fracture. B. Closed reduction and hip pinning.

Femur
Greater Trochanter

Anatomy
-"Traction" apophysis

Clinical Diagnosis
-May accompany hip dislocation

Radiologic Diagnosis
-May be a fracture through the ossification center (type 7 injury)
-May be a fracture with variable displacement, through the physis (type 1 injury)

Recommended Treatment
-Traction if concomitant hip dislocation
-Progressive weight-bearing
-May require open reduction when displaced

Complications
-Premature epiphyseodesis can lead to elongated femoral neck

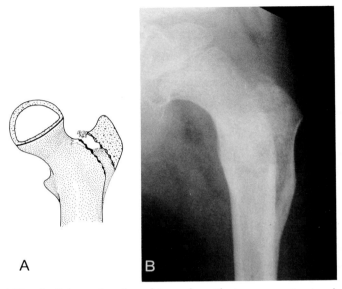

Figure 165. A. Schematic of avulsion of cartilaginous greater trochanter. B. Radiograph showing extensive subperiosteal bone.

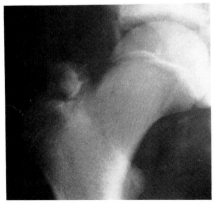

Figure 166. Type 7 injury through greater trochanter.

Femur
Lesser Trochanter

Anatomy
-Avulsion injury of attachment of iliopsoas tendon

Clinical Diagnosis
-Pain in groin or inner thigh
-Often seen in adolescent sports (especially sprinting)

Radiologic Diagnosis
-Avulsion of small portion of lesser trochanter
-Cannot be diagnosed if only cartilage is avulsed (look for callus at two to three weeks)

Recommended treatment
-Crutches, progressive weight bearing
-Discontinue athletic activity until healed (three to six weeks); must have progressive muscular rehabilitation

Complications
-Excessive bone formation, especially when there is chronic injury
-Chronic pain

Reference

Wilson MJ, Michele AA, Jacobson, EW: Isolated fracture of the lesser trochanter. J Bone Joint Surg 21:776, 1939.

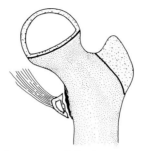

Figure 167. Schematic of avulsion of the lesser trochanter.

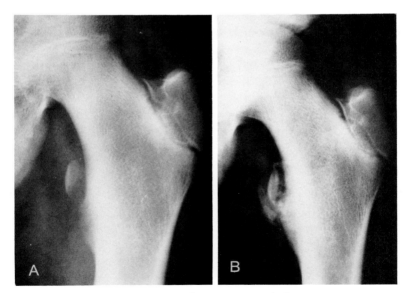

Figure 168. A. Early injury. B. Ossification 11 weeks later.

Femur
Subtrochanteric Fracture

Figures 169–170

Anatomy
-Unstable injury at or below level of lesser trochanter
-Periosteal sleeve may be partially intact in younger child, introducing a degree of intrinsic stability

Clinical Diagnosis
-Painful hip

Radiologic Diagnosis
-Assess anatomic characteristics of fracture, degree of abduction of proximal fragment

Recommended Treatment
-Traction
-Open reduction if alignment cannot be maintained (especially in older child)

Complications
-Malunion
-Late slipped capital femoral epiphysis

References

Ireland DCR, Fisher RL: Subtrochanteric fractures of the femur in children. Clin Orthop 110:157, 1975.

Ogden JA, Gossling HR, Southwick WO: Slipped capital femoral epiphysis following ipsilateral femoral fracture. Clin Orthop 110:167, 1975.

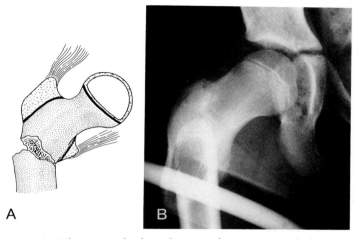

Figure 169. A. Schematic of subtrochanteric fracture. B. Radiology.

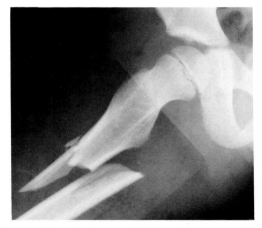

Figure 170. The muscle pulls flex and abduct the proximal fragment. Accordingly the distal fragment must be aligned in traction.

Femur
Diaphysis

Anatomy
-Minimal displacement in infant, young child
-Greater tendency to overriding after two years
-Femur normally has mild anterolateral bowing

Clinical Diagnosis
-Swollen, painful thigh
-Careful assessment of neurovascular injury
-Monitor blood loss into thigh

Radiologic Diagnosis
-Assess extent of overriding, angulation
-Assess hip for concomitant dislocation

Recommended Treatment
-Allow overriding of approximately 1 to 2 cm
-Traction with emphasis on longitudinal and rotational alignment
-Early cast, especially in younger children

Complications
-Overgrowth very common in two- to ten-year range
-Vascular injury
-Damage to trochanteric physis if intramedullary nail used

References

Brouwer KJ, Molenaar JC, Van Linge B: Rotational deformities after femoral shaft fractures in childhood. Acta Orthop Scand 52:81–89, 1981.

Gross RH, Davidson R, Sullivan JA, Peeples RE, Hufft R: Cast brace management of the femoral shaft fracture in children and young adults. J Pediatr Orthop 3:572–582, 1983.

Miller PR, Welch MC: The hazards of tibia pin replacement in 90-90 skeletal traction. Clin Orthop 135:97–100, 1978.

Shapiro F: Fractures of the femoral shaft in children. The overgrowth phenomenon. Acta Orthop Scand 52:649–655, 1981.

Ziv I, Blackburn N, Rang M: Femoral intramedullary nailing in the growing child. J Trauma 24:432–434, 1984.

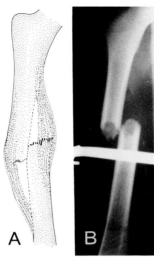

Figure 171. A. Schematic of diaphyseal femoral fracture. B. Typical overriding present in a seven-year-old.

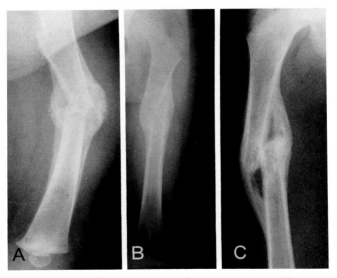

Figure 172. A. Typical callus at seven weeks in a one-year-old. B. More limited callus with remodeling nine months after an overriding femoral diaphysis fracture in a seven-year-old. C. Extensive subperiosteal new bone in continuous periosteal sleeve, despite overriding.

Femur
Distal Metaphysis

Anatomy
-Often a torus injury
-Comminution

Clinical Diagnosis
-Pain, swelling above knee

Radiologic Diagnosis
-Try to evaluate changes in varus/valgus

Recommended Treatment
-Closed, with or without traction
-Muscular attachment may angulate the distal fragment posteriorly
-Angular deformity

Complications
-Watch for physeal injury several months later

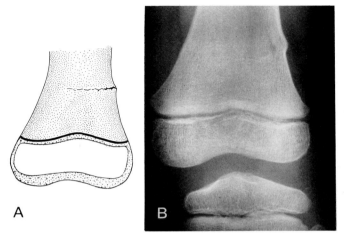

Figure 173. A. Schematic of metaphyseal fracture. B. Torus injury of distal metaphysis.

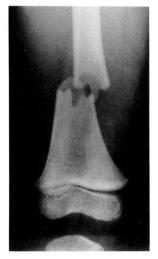

Figure 174. Complete metaphyseal fracture.

Femur
Distal Physis

Anatomy
-Major contributor to leg length (40%)

Clinical Diagnosis
-Pain, swelling above knee
-Possible hemarthrosis or sympathetic knee effusion

Radiologic Diagnosis
-Assess pattern
-May require stress view

Recommended Treatment
-Closed reduction of types 1,2 (internal fixation of type 2 may be indicated if unstable)
-Types 3 and 4 require open reduction, internal fixation

Complications
-Growth arrest
-Progressive angular deformity of growth arrest is eccentric
-Shortening if growth arrest is central or complete

Reference
Riseborough EJ, Barrett IR, Shapiro F: Growth disturbance following distal femoral physeal fracture-separations. J Bone Joint Surg 65A:885–893, 1983.

178   POCKET GUIDE TO PEDIATRIC FRACTURES

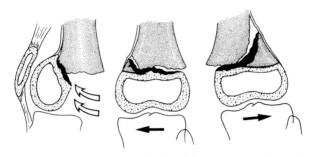

Figure 175. Schematic of type 1 and 2 distal femoral growth mechanism injury.

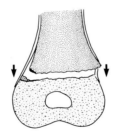

TYPE 1–INFANCY

Figure 176. Schematic of type 1 injury in infancy or child abuse.

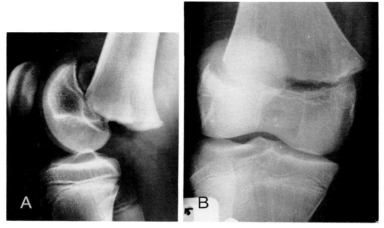

Figure 177. A. Typical anteriorly displaced type 1 distal femoral lesion. B. Initial attempt at reduction. The valgus angulation still needs to be corrected.

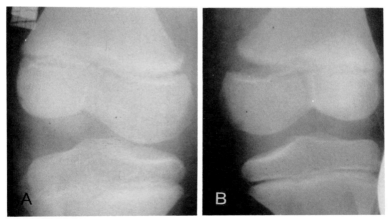

Figure 178. A. Questionable injury in adolescent with knee injury and hemarthrosis. B. Stress film revealed a type 3 injury of one femoral condyle.

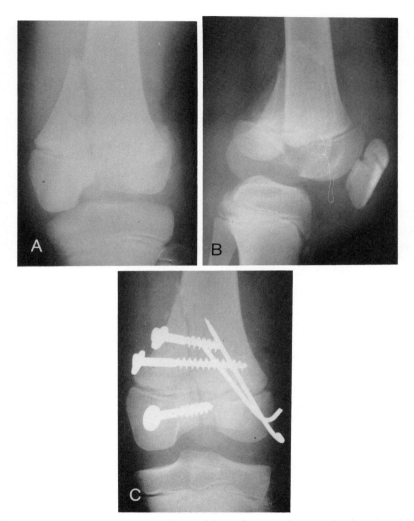

Figure 179. A, B. Anteroposterior and lateral views show multiple injuries to the distal femur and patella. C. Postreduction with internal fixation.

Knee
Osteochondral Injury

Anatomy
-Usually referred to as osteochondritis dissecans
-Generally affects medial condyle near intercondylar notch
-Osteochondral type 7 injury

Clinical Diagnosis
-May be acute injury
-Chronic knee pain more common
-May have effusion

Radiologic Diagnosis
-Assess displacement of fragment
-May require special views, arthrography

Recommended Treatment
-If undisplaced: nonweight-bearing with at least two to three weeks of
 knee immobilization
-If displaced, reduction and fixation (may be done arthroscopically)
-Loose fragment may have to be removed and defect drilled to en-
 courage vascularization and development of fibrocartilage

Complications
-Non-union
-Disruption of articular surface

Reference
Green WT, Banks HH:Osteochondritis dissecans in children. J Bone Joint Surg 35A:26,
  1953.

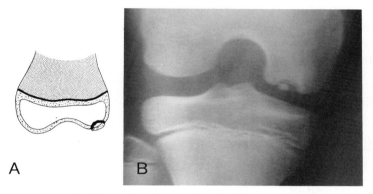

Figure 180. A. Schematic of osteochondral fracture. B. Typical lesion.

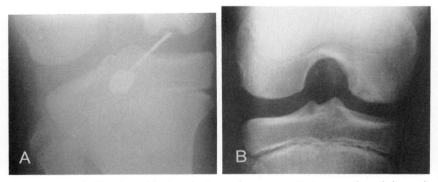

Figure 181. A. Fixation of lesion during arthroscopy. A pin was placed through this. B. Six months later the lesion is healed and the pin has been removed.

Knee Dislocation

Anatomy
-Medial, lateral ligaments not usually disrupted
-Cruciate ligament injury more likely
-Neurovascular structures relatively fixed just above femoral condyles, increasing susceptibility to injury

Clinical Diagnosis
-Carefully examine neurovascular status

Radiologic Diagnosis
-Look for accompanying fractures

Recommended Treatment
-Closed reduction
-Immobilization for four to six weeks

Complications
-Vascular disruption
-Compartment syndrome
-Ligamentous laxity

Reference
Gartland JJ, Brenner JH: Traumatic dislocations in the lower extremity in children. Orthop Clin North Am 7:687, 1976.

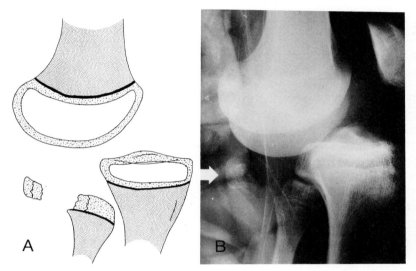

Figure 182. A. Schematic of knee dislocation. B. Complete posterior dislocation of distal femur. Note that the proximal fibula has a type 3 growth mechanism fracture.

Knee
Patellar Dislocation

Anatomy
-Usually lateral displacement, with disruption of medial soft tissues

Clinical Diagnosis
-Patella located along lateral condyle

Radiologic Diagnosis
-Abnormal patellar location
-Look for associated fractures from condyles or patella

Recommended Treatment
-Closed reduction
-Reassess for fractures after reduction
-Three to four weeks of extension immobilization
-Progressive rehabilitation
-Accompanying fracture may require fixation

Complications
-Chronic instability
-Osteochondral fragment

References

McManus F, Rang M, Heslin DJ: Acute dislocation of the patella in children. The natural history. Clin Orthop 139:88–91, 1979.

Rorabeck CH, Bobechko WP: Acute dislocation of the patella with osteochondral fracture. J Bone Joint Surg 58B:237–240, 1976.

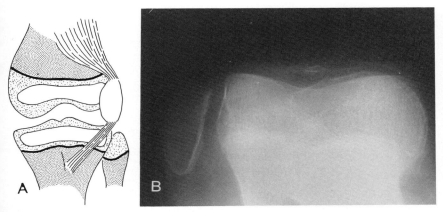

Figure 183. A. Schematic of patellar dislocation. B. Radiograph of complete dislocation.

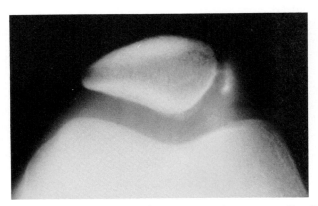

Figure 184. Typical medial margin fracture complicating patellar dislocation.

Knee
Patellar Subluxation

Figure 185

Anatomy
-Movement of patella varies from longitudinal axis

Clinical Diagnosis
-Apprehension when examiner attempts to lateralize the patella

Radiologic Diagnosis
-Decreased height of lateral condyle and asymmetric shape of patella in "sunrise" views

Recommended Treatment
-Quadriceps rehabilitation
-Rarely requires surgery prior to skeletal maturation

Complications
-Chronic subluxation
-Chronic pain

Reference
Cross MJ, Waldrop J: The patellar index as a guide to the understanding and diagnosis of patellofemoral instability Clin Orthop 110:174, 1975.

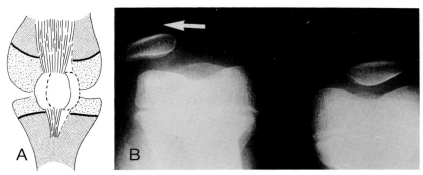

Figure 185. A. Schematic of patellar subluxation. B. "Sunrise" view showing lateralization of patella (arrow).

Knee
Collateral Ligaments

Anatomy
-Usually a chondro-osseous disruption, rather than ligament injury prior to skeletal maturity
-However, true disruption within ligament may occur

Clinical Diagnosis
-Pain and tenderness over ligament, especially over chondro-osseous attachment
-Joint effusion, bleeding

Radiologic Diagnosis
-Small avulsion fracture

Recommended Treatment
-Closed, with three to four weeks of immobilization until fracture heals

Complications
-Chronic ligamentous laxity
-Non-union of avulsion fracture

References

Bertin KC, Cable EM: Ligament injuries associated with physeal fractures about the knee. Clin Orthop 177:188–195, 1983.
Clanton TO, DeLee JC, Sanders, B, Neidre A: Knee ligament injuries in children. J Bone Joint Surg 61A:1195–1201, 1979.

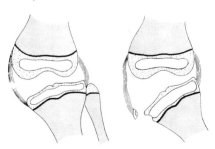

Figure 186. Schematics of collateral ligament injury showing ligament disruption (left) versus osteochondral avulsion (right).

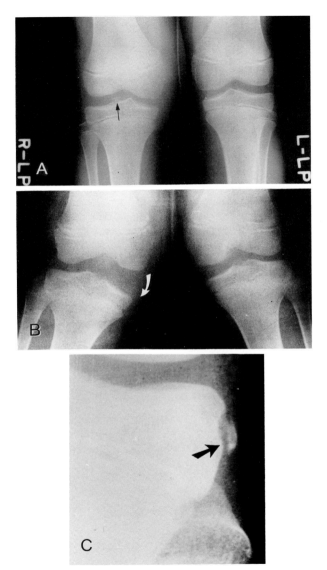

Figure 187. A. Apparent tibial spine injury in unstressed view. B. However, ligament injury was evident in stress film. C. Osteochondral avulsion of collateral ligament from the proximal tibial epiphysis.

Knee
Patellar Fracture

Anatomy
-Variable amount of cartilage

Clinical Diagnosis
-Painful patella
-Knee effusion

Radiologic Diagnosis
-Most frequent fractures are in mid-portion
-Bipartite patella, while normally considered a radiologic variant, may also be an acute or chronic injury

Recommended Treatment
-Closed, if not displaced
-Open reduction, tension band wiring

Complications
-Non-union
-Elongated patella

Reference

Ogden JA, McCarthy SM, Jokl P: The painful bipartite patella J Pediatr Orthop 2:263–269, 1982.

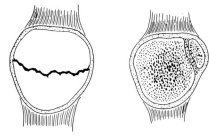

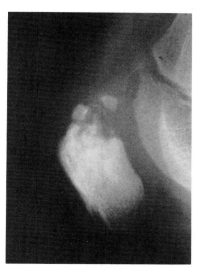

Figure 188. Schematics of undisplaced patellar fracture (left; also see Fig. 179) and bipartite patella (right).

Figure 189. Patellar fracture.

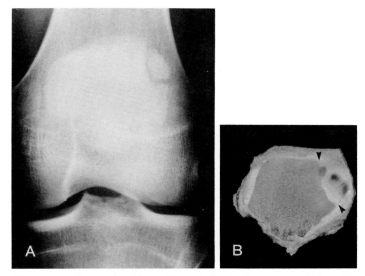

Figure 190. A. Radiograph of bipartite patella. B. Specimen of bipartite patella showing cartilaginous continuity.

Knee
Distal Patella

Anatomy

-Tension failure, either acute or chronic, at chondro-osseous junction
-Chronic failure is usually referred to as Sinding-Larsen-Johansson injury
 (analogous to Osgood-Schlatter's lesion at other end of patellar tendon)

Clinical Diagnosis

-Pain at lower (inferior) part of patella

Radiologic Diagnosis

-May be a very thin piece of bone at the distal chondro-osseous junction
 ("sleeve" fracture)
-May be a retrospective diagnosis, especially in the chronic injury

Recommended Treatment

-Immobilization in cylinder cast for at least three weeks
-Progressive rehabilitation

Complications

-Elongation of patella
-Chronic pain

References

Houghton GR, Ackroyd CE. Sleeve fractures of the patella in children. J Bone Joint Surg.
    61B:165–168, 1979.
Medlar RC, Lyne ED: Sinding-Larsen-Johansson disease J Bone Joint Surg 60A:1113, 1978.

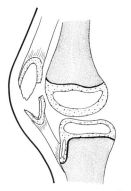

Figure 191. Schematic of sleeve fracture.

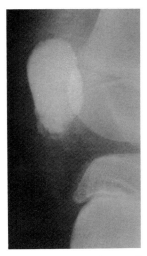

Figure 193. An early Sinding-Larsen-Johannson lesion of the distal pole of the patella. This is analogous to the Osgood-Schlatter's injury at the other end of the patellar tendon.

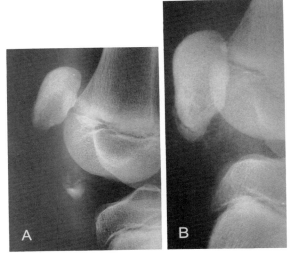

Figure 192. A. Displaced sleeve fracture. B. Three weeks after open reduction.

Knee
Meniscal Injury

Anatomy
-Vascularity decreases with age, but is retained peripherally
-Discoid meniscus may be a lateral congenital variation (but it can be damaged)

Clinical Diagnosis
-Similar to adult: locking, effusion, sense of instability
-Discoid lateral meniscus may "pop" with flexion/extension

Radiologic Diagnosis
-Arthrography
-Possible role of magnetic resonance imaging

Recommended Treatment
-Repair whenever possible, rather than excision
-Recontour the discoid lateral meniscus into a C-shape

Complications
-Arthritis
-Derangement of knee mechanics

References

Clark CR, Ogden JA: Development of the menisci of the human knee Joint. Morphological changes and their potential role in childhood meniscal injury. J Bone Joint Surg. 65A:538–547, 1983.

Mangione M, Pizzutillo PD, Peoples AB, Schweizer PA: Meniscectomy in children: a long-term follow up study. Am J Sports Med 11:111–115, 1983.

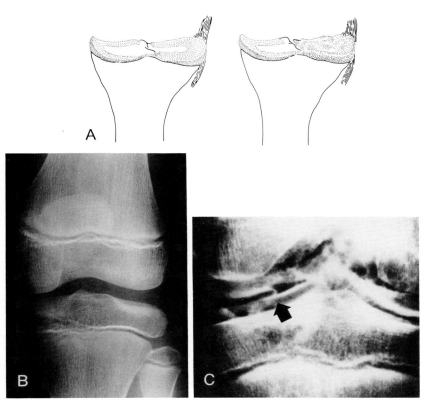

Figure 194. A. Schematic of normal (left) and discoid (right) menisci. B. Typical widened, sclerotic lateral compartment. C. Arthrogram showing torn discoid lateral meniscus (arrow).

Tibia/Fibula
Tibial Spines

Anatomy
-Analogue of cruciate ligament injury in the adult

Clinical Diagnosis
-Swollen knee
-Motion restriction
-Hemarthrosis

Radiologic Diagnosis
-Lateral view is essential to show anteroposterior extent of the injury and the degree of displacement

Recommended Treatment
-Closed if undisplaced
-Open if displaced

Complications
-Chronic cruciate ligament insufficiency
-Non-union with or without pain

References

DeLee JC, Curtis R: Anterior cruciate ligament insufficiencies in children. Clin Orthop 172:112–118, 1983.

Meyers M, McKeever F: Fractures of the intercondylar eminence of the tibia. J Bone Joint Surg 52A:1677–1684, 1970.

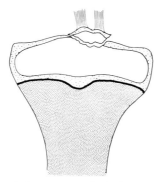

Figure 195. Schematic of disruption of tibial spines with attached cruciate ligaments.

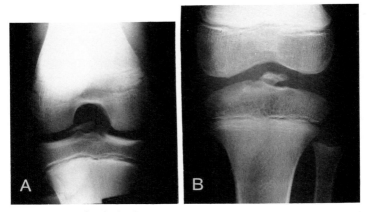

Figure 196. A. Avulsed tibial spine. B. Non-union present three months after original knee injury.

Tibia/Fibula
Proximal Epiphysis

Anatomy
-Infrequently injured area due to morphology, especially anterior over-
  lap of the tuberosity

Clinical Diagnosis
-Swelling, tenderness below the knee
-Sympathetic knee effusion
-Assess the neurovascular status

Radiologic Diagnosis
-Assess degree of displacement

Recommended Treatment
-Closed reduction, types 1 and 2
-Open reduction, types 3 and 4

Complications
-Neurovascular injury
-Growth damage
-Angulation

References

Burkhart SS, Peterson HA: Fractures of the proximal tibial epiphysis. J Bone Joint Surg
  61A:996–1002, 1979.
Shelton WR, Canale ST: Fractures of the tibia through the proximal tibial epiphyseal
  cartilage. J Bone Joint Surg 61A:167–173, 1979.

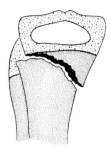

Figure 197. Schematic of proximal tibial physeal/epiphyseal injury.

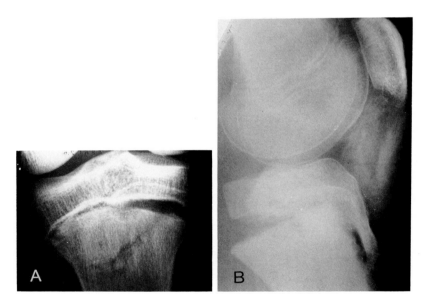

Figure 198. A. Type 2 injury. B. Type 1 injury.

Tibia/Fibula
Tibial Tuberosity

Figure 199

Anatomy
-Apophysis
-Tends to occur in adolescence

Clinical Diagnosis
-Painful prominent tuberosity

Radiologic Diagnosis
-Variable displacement
-Assess extension into joint

Recommended Treatment
-Closed reduction when undisplaced (but watch closely for changed position within the first two weeks)
-Open reduction whenever displaced

Complications
-Avulsion after fixation
-Intra-articular damage

Reference

Ogden JA, Tross RB, Murphy MJ: Fractures of the tibial tuberosity in adolescents. J Bone Joint Surg 62A:205–215, 1980.

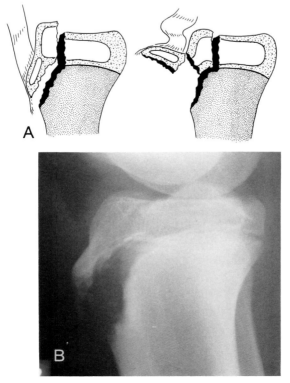

Figure 199. A. Schematics of tibial tuberosity injuries. B. Appearance of avulsed fracture of the tibial tuberosity.

Tibia/Fibula Osgood-Schlatter's Lesion

Figures 200–201

Anatomy
-Chronic stress injury
-Infrequently acute

Clinical Diagnosis
-Painful tibial tuberosity

Radiologic Diagnosis
-Irregular ossification within the tuberosity
-Late stage may be associated with ossicle formation

Recommended Treatment
-Immobilization for one to three weeks until pain gone
-Progressive quadriceps strengthening
-Rarely lateral retinacular release or resection of ossicle(s) indicated

Complications
-Enlargement of the tuberosity
-Chronic pain due to ossicles, chronic motion

References

Mital M, Matza RA: The unresolved Osgood-Schlatter's condition. Orthop Trans 2:71, 1978.

Ogden JA: The Osgood-Schlatter's injury. J Pediatr Orthop, submitted for publication.

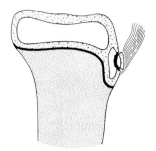

Figure 200. Schematic of Osgood-Schlatter's lesion.

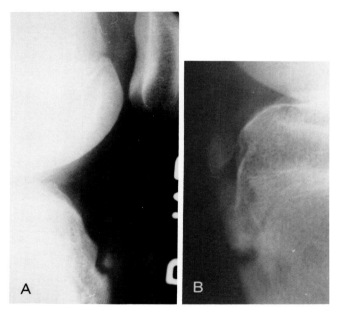

Figure 201. Typical chronic Osgood-Schlatter injuries seven months (A) and two years (B) after symptom onset, but without immobilization. These are nonunions.

Tibia/Fibula
Proximal Fibula

Figure 202

Anatomy
-Attachment of biceps
-Proximity of peroneal nerve

Clinical Diagnosis
-Pain over proximal fibula
-Assess peroneal nerve function

Radiologic Diagnosis
-Assess extent of displacement

Recommended Treatment
-Closed reduction if undisplaced
-Open reduction if displaced or if neurologic findings are present

Complications
-Peroneal palsy
-Growth deformity

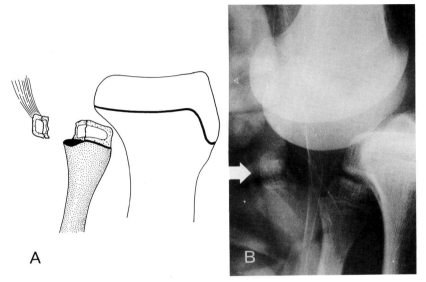

Figure 202. A. Schematic of proximal fibular injury. B. Radiograph of injury (arrow) accompanying a knee dislocation.

Tibia/Fibula
Proximal Fibula
Dislocation

Anatomy
-Proximity of peroneal nerve
-Variability of morphology of tibiofibular joint

Clinical Diagnosis
-Painful anterolateral mass

Radiologic Diagnosis
-Disruption of proximal tibiofibular joint
-May require oblique views

Recommended Treatment
-Closed reduction

Complications
-Peroneal nerve dysfunction
-Chronic pain and instability

Reference

Ogden JA: Subluxation and dislocation of the proximal tibiofibular joint. J Bone Joint Surg, 56A:145–154, 1974

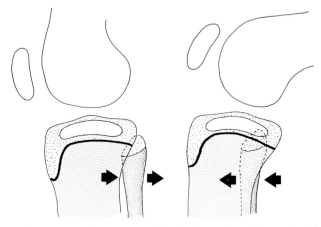

Figure 203. Schematic of proximal tibiofibular subluxation and dislocation.

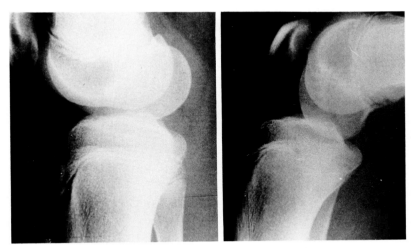

Figure 204. Normal (right) versus anterior dislocation (left).

Tibia/Fibula
Proximal Metaphysis

Anatomy
-Variability of vascularity between medial and lateral segments

Clinical Diagnosis
-Pain, swelling distal to knee

Radiologic Diagnosis
-Usually an incomplete tibial fracture (fibula usually not injured)

Recommended Treatment
-Closed, with three point pressure to maintain alignment

Complications
-*Progressive* valgus deformity (may occur within first few weeks and is non-progressive after six to nine months)

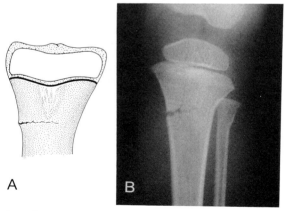

Figure 205. A. Schematic of proximal metaphyseal tibial fracture B. Typical injury pattern.

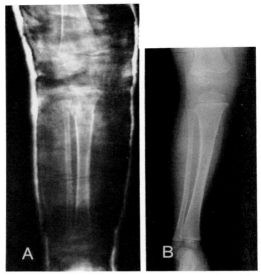

Figure 206. A. Fracture of metaphysis with no angular deformity two weeks after injury. B. Valgus angulation twelve weeks later.

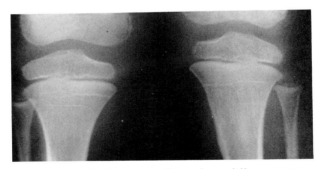

Figure 207. Harris growth slow-down lines show differences in growth rates medially versus laterally in a valgus deformity of the left tibia (contrast with similar line on the right).

References

Balthazar DA, Pappas AM: Acquired valgus deformity of the tibia in children. J Pediatr Orthop 4:538–541, 1984.

Jackson DW, Cozen L: Genu valgum as a complication of proximal tibial metaphyseal fractures in children. J Bone Joint Surg 53A:1571–1578, 1971.

Tibia/Fibula Diaphysis

Anatomy
-Increased thickening of the cortex is a factor in simple versus comminuted fracture
-Extent of osteon formation a factor in toddler's fracture

Clinical Diagnosis
-Painful, swollen lower leg
-Assess compartment pressure, neurovascular status

Radiologic Diagnosis
-Assess fracture pattern, degree of overriding, shortening

Recommended Treatment
-Closed
-Maintain length as much as possible

Complications
-Increased possibility of delayed union or non-union as child matures into adolescence.

Reference

Hansen BA, Greiff J, Bergmann F: Fractures of the tibia in children. Acta Orthop Scand 47:448–453, 1976.

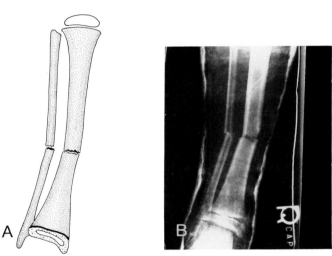

Figure 208. A. Schematic of diaphyseal tibiofibular fractures. B. Typical fracture.

Tibia/Fibula
Toddler's Fracture

Figure 209

Anatomy

-Occurs as child is first walking, when diaphysis still has considerable woven rather than osteon bone
-May involve either tibia or fibula

Clinical Diagnosis

-Pain in leg
-Limping

Radiologic Diagnosis

-Often not possible acutely
-Look for bowing of the fibula

Recommended Treatment

-Cast immobilization

Complications

-Limping

Reference

Dunbar JS, Owen HF, Nogrady MB, McLeese R: Obscure tibial fracture of infants-the toddler's fracture. J Can Assoc Radiol 15:136–144, 1964.

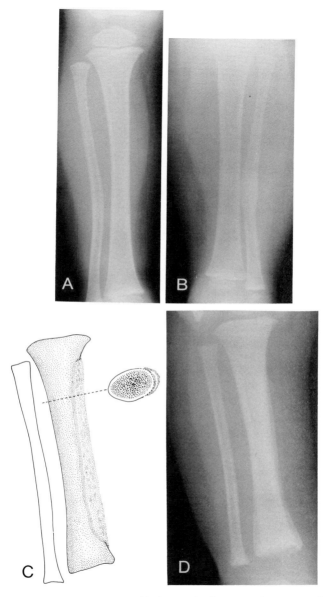

Figure 209. A. Typical bowing of fibula. B. Thickening subperiosteal new bone along fibula. C. Schematic. D. Subperiosteal bone in tibial toddler's fracture six weeks after onset of limping.

Tibia/Fibula
Distal Metaphysis

Figure 210

Anatomy
-Variability of metaphyseal cortex

Clinical Diagnosis
-Painful above the ankle

Radiologic Diagnosis
-Assess displacement, comminution
-Fibula may have severe angulation

Recommended Treatment
-Closed reduction (may require rotational manipulation to correct fibular angulation)

Complications
-Angular deformity

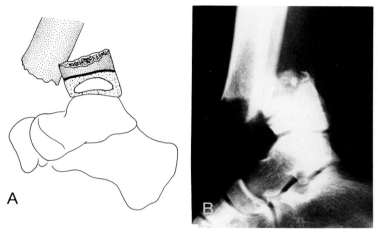

Figure 210. A. Schematic of distal metaphyseal fracture. B. Radiograph.

Tibia/Fibula Distal Epiphysis (Types 1 and 2)

Figure 211

Anatomy
-Relatively planar growth plate
-May displace with rotation only

Clinical Diagnosis
-Painful, swollen ankle

Radiologic Diagnosis
-Normal irregularity of physis just above malleolus should not be misinterpreted as a fracture
-Must distinguish type 2 from more complex injuries
-Be wary of pure rotational displacement

Recommended Treatment
-Closed reduction

Complications
-Growth arrest

References

Dias LS, Tachdjian MO: Physeal injuries of the ankle in children. Clin Orthop 136:230, 1978.
Lovell ES: An unusual rotatory injury of the ankle. J Bone Joint Surg 50A:222–223, 1968.

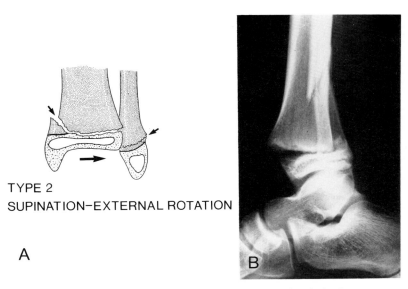

TYPE 2
SUPINATION–EXTERNAL ROTATION

A

B

Figure 211. A. Schematic of type 2 injury. B. Type 2 distal tibial injury.

Tibia/Fibula
Distal Epiphysis (Triplane)

Figures 212–213

Anatomy
-Combination of type 3 and 4 injuries

Clinical Diagnosis
-Swollen, painful ankle

Radiologic Diagnosis
-Anteroposterior/lateral will not completely reveal morphology of injury
-May require CT imaging for complete delineation

Recommended Treatment
-Open reduction

Complications
-Growth arrest

References

Spiegel PG, Mast JW, Cooperman DR, Laros GS: Triplane fractures of the distal tibial epiphysis. Clin Orthop 188:74–89, 1984.

Spiegel PG, Cooperman DR, Laros GS: Epiphyseal fractures of the distal ends of the tibia and fibula. J Bone Joint Surg 60A:1046–1050, 1978.

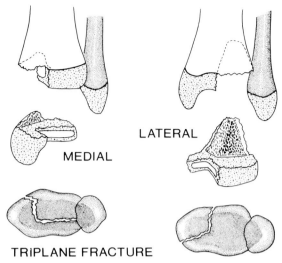

MEDIAL

LATERAL

TRIPLANE FRACTURE

Figure 212. A. Schematic of triplane fractures.

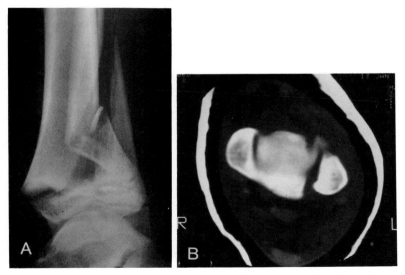

Figure 213. A. Triplane fracture. B. CT scan showing articular disruption.

Tibia/Fibula
Distal Epiphysis (Tillaux)

Anatomy
-Relates to pattern of closure of physis: medial side closes before lateral
 side

Clinical Diagnosis
-Painful, swollen ankle

Radiologic Diagnosis
-May require oblique or mortise view to delineate extent of injury
-CT scan may delineate degree of separation

Recommended Treatment
-Closed when fracture is undisplaced
-Open, with fixation, if displacement interrupts joint congruity

Complications
-Arthritis

Reference

Kleiger B, Mankin HJ: Fracture of the lateral portion of the distal tibial epiphysis. J Bone
 Joint Surg 46A:25, 1964.

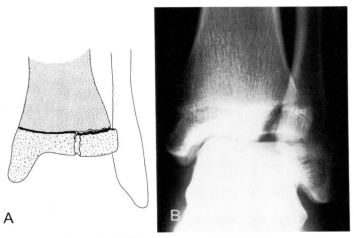

Figure 214. A. Schematic of Tillaux fracture. B. Typical appearance.

Tibia/Fibula
Distal Epiphysis (Malleoli)

Anatomy
-Type 3 or 4 injury
-Type 7 injury
-Malleolar

Clinical Diagnosis
-Painful, swollen over involved malleolus

Radiologic Diagnosis
-Must assess extent of displacement

Recommended Treatment
-Usually require open reduction
-Type 7 may be treated closed when undisplaced

Complications
-Growth arrest
-Angular deformity

Reference

Kling TF, Bright RW, Hensinger RN: Distal tibial physeal fractures in children that may require open reduction. J Bone Joint Surg 66A:647–657, 1984

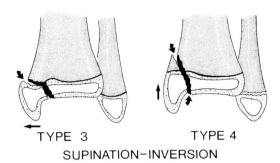

TYPE 3   TYPE 4

SUPINATION–INVERSION

Figure 215. Schematic of types 3 and 4 injuries.

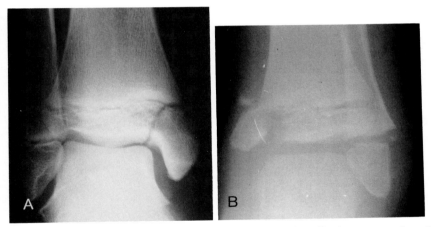

Figure 216. A. Undisplaced type 3 injury of medial malleolus. B. Displaced type 4 injury with concomitant type 2 injury of the lateral malleolus.

Foot
Puncture Wounds

Figure 217

Anatomy
-May extend to skeletal components or joints

Clinical Diagnosis
-Small puncture wound may be all that is readily evident

Radiologic Diagnosis
-Look for foreign material (e.g., wood, metal)
-Look for osseous cortical injury

Recommended Treatment
-Antibiotic coverage
-Debridement when indicated

Complications
-Osteomyelitis
-Septic arthritis
-Abscess

References

Brand RA, Black H: Pseudomonas osteomyelitis following puncture wounds in children. J Bone Joint Surg 56A:1637, 1974.

Johansson PH: Pseudomonas infections of the foot following puncture wounds in children. JAMA 204:262, 1968.

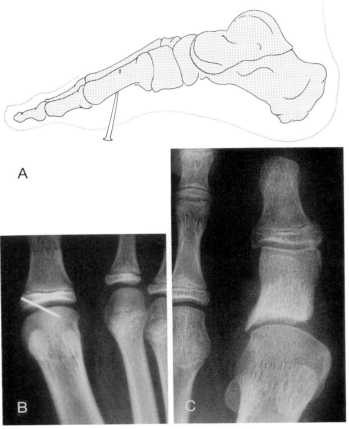

Figure 217. A. Schematic of puncture wound. B. Pin penetration into joint and bone. C. Shortened phalanx of hallux due to osteomyelitis (*Pseudomonas*) following seemingly innocuous puncture wound.

Foot
Talus

Anatomy
-Vascularity changes with chondro-osseous maturation
-Accessory ossification potential in posterior region (os trigonum)

Clinical Diagnosis
-Pain with ankle motion; swollen in ankle region

Radiologic Diagnosis
-Neck fracture
-Osteochondritis of articular margin
-Os trigonum: acute vs. chronic

Recommended Treatment
-Neck fracture—closed vs. open depends upon displacement
-Osteochondritis—immobilization
-Os trigonum—immobilization

Complications
-Ischemic necrosis
-Chronic joint pain

References

Canale ST, Belding RH: Osteochondral lesions of the talus. J Bone Joint Surg 62A:97–102, 1980

Letts RM, Gibeaut D: Fracture of the neck of the talus in children. Foot Ankle 1:74–77, 1980

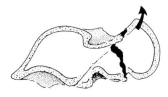

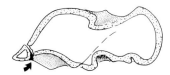

Figure 218. Schematic of fracture of the talar neck (top) and os trigonum (bottom).

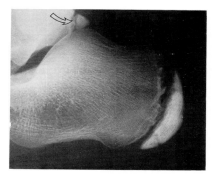

Figure 220. Os trigonum (arrow) in patient with Sever's diseases.

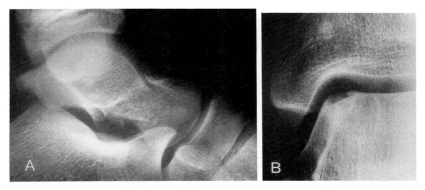

Figure 219. A. Typical talar neck fracture in an 11-year-old. B. Typical talar osteochondritic lesion.

Foot
Calcaneus

Figures 221–222

Anatomy
-Variability of secondary ossification in apophysis

Clinical Diagnosis
-Pain in heel

Radiologic Diagnosis
-Look at fracture line in body
-Variable sclerosis of apophysis difficult to diagnose (possibility of Sever's disease)

Recommended Treatment
-Closed whenever possible

Complications
-Growth arrest
-Subtalar arthritis

References

Matteri R, Frymoyer J: Fractures of the calcaneus in young children. J Bone Joint Surg 55A:1091, 1973.

Schmidt TL, Weiner DS: Calcaneal fractures in children. An evaluation of the nature of the injury in 56 children. Clin Orthop 171:150–155, 1982.

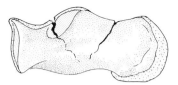

Figure 221. Schematic of typical fracture lines.

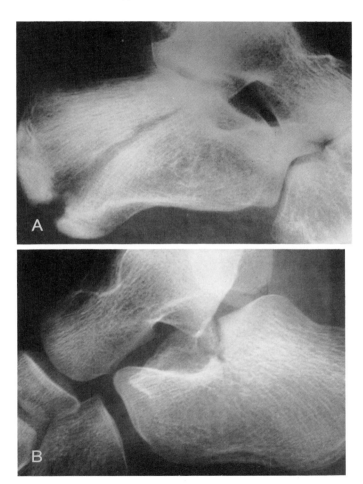

Figure 222. A. Fracture through body of calcaneus, but without subtalar involvement. B. Fracture involving subtalar joints.

Foot
Tarsal Coalition

Figure 223

Anatomy
-Types of bars vary: calcaneonavicular most common

Clinical Diagnosis
-Often present as acute onset of pain

Radiologic Diagnosis
-Often require special views

Recommended Treatment
-Immobilization
-Orthotics
-Bridge resection

Complications
-Recurrent pain

Reference
Richards RR, Evans JG, McGoey PF: Fracture of a calcaneonavicular bar: a complication of tarsal coalition. A case report. Clin Orthop 185:220–221, 1984.

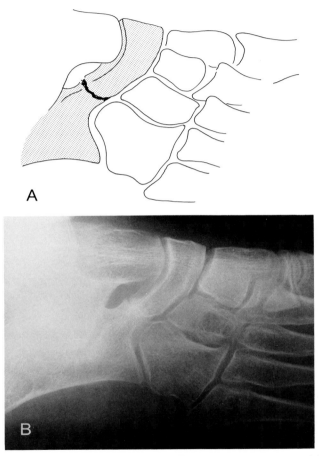

Figure 223. A. Schematic of tarsal coalition. B. Mature, painful coalition between calcaneus and tarsal navicular.

Foot
Navicula

Anatomy
-Variability in ossification

Clinical Diagnosis
-Pain in dorsum of midfoot

Radiologic Diagnosis
-Irregularity of ossification (osteochondritis)
-Presence of accessory navicular
-Bone scan useful

Recommended Treatment
-Immobilization
-Excision of accessory navicular if chronically painful

Complications
-Pes planus (painful)

Reference

Lawson JP, Ogden JA, Sella E, Barwick KW: The painful accessory navicular. Skel Radiol 12:250–262, 1984.

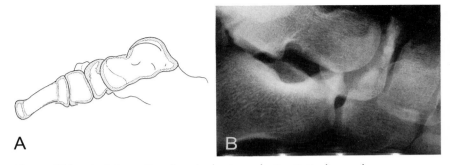

Figure 224. A. Schematic of navicular irregularity. B. Radiograph.

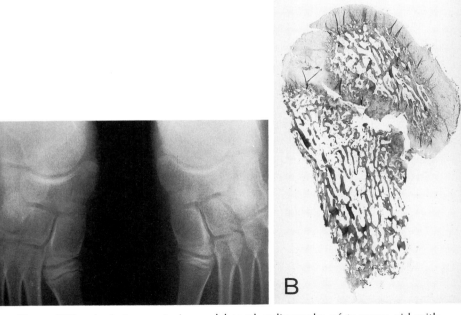

Figure 225. A. Anteroposterior and lateral radiographs of teenage girl with painful flat feet and accessory tarsal naviculars. B. Histologic section showing fracture between the main and accessory ossification centers. This is a stress fracture.

Foot
Metatarsals

Anatomy
-Proximal physis/epiphysis in first metatarsal
-Distal physis/epiphysis in other metatarsals
-Shaft fractures more common than physeal

Clinical Diagnosis
-Painful, swollen; especially on dorsum of the foot

Radiologic Diagnosis
-Variable displacement of metatarsals in shaft fracture
-Angulation of distal physeal fractures

Recommended Treatment
-Closed reduction

Complications
-Chronic pain
-Growth arrest (especially in first metatarsal) leading to short bone

Reference
Wiley JJ: Tarsometatarsal joint injuries in children. J Pediatr Orthop 1:255–260, 1981.

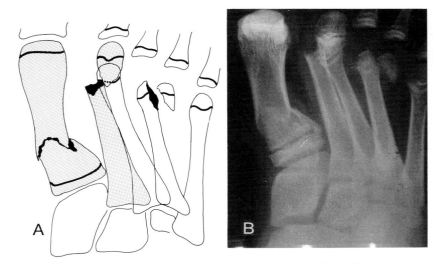

Figure 226. A. Schematic of metatarsal fractures. B. Radiograph.

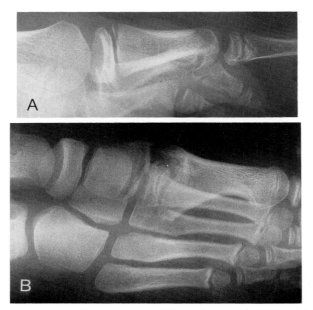

Figure 227. A. Undisplaced type 2 growth mechanism fracture of the proximal first metatarsal. B. Growth damage following such a fracture.

Foot
Proximal Fifth Metatarsal

Figure 228

Anatomy
-Apophyseal injury
-Peroneal musculature attachment

Clinical Diagnosis
-Point tenderness, swelling over proximal end of metatarsal

Radiologic Diagnosis
-Do not confuse with secondary ossification center

Recommended Treatment
-Closed reduction, immobilization

Complications
-Non-union

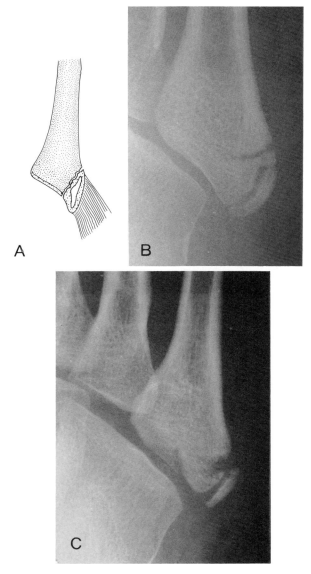

Figure 228. A. Schematic. B, C. Radiographs of undisplaced (B) and displaced (C) fractures.

Foot
Phalanges

Anatomy
-Most common in great toe
-Small bones minimize injury in other four toes

Clinical Diagnosis
-Painful, swollen toe

Radiologic Diagnosis
-Assess physeal injury, especially in stubbing injury

Recommended Treatment
-Closed reduction when necessary
-Antibiotics if open nail or pulp space injury

Complications
-Angulation
-Growth arrest
-Nail injury
-Infection

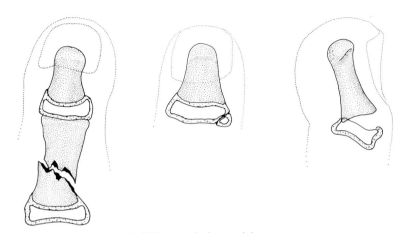

Figure 229. Schematic of different phalangeal fractures.

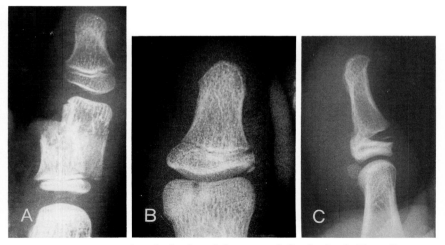

Figure 230. A. Angulated, displaced fracture of diaphysis. B. Type 7 osteochondral (ligament analogue) fracture. C. Type 2 physeal injury.

INDEX

Acromion, 58
Anesthesia, in fracture treatment, 8, 9, 24
Ankle, fractures of, 216–225
Arteriography, in fracture complications, 19, 20
Arthrography, 1, 17
Articular cartilage, fracture of, 4, 30, 32
Athletic injury(ies), 22, 50
Atlantoaxial joint, dislocation of, 140, 141
Atlas, fracture of, 138, 139

Battered-child syndrome, 24, 52
Bayonet apposition, in fracture treatment, 10
Bennett's fracture, 116, 117
Bipartite patella, 192, 193
Birth injury, 44, 72
Bladder, injury to, 152
Bone scanning, 18, 46, 51
Bowing, 5
Burn(s), 11, 36

Calcaneus, injury of, 230, 231
Callus, 10, 46, 56
Capitellum (capitulum), 74
Carpus, injury of, 112, 113
Cervical spine, 138–147
Child abuse, 24, 52
Chondroepiphysis, anatomy of, 4
Clavicle, 44, 54–59
Collateral ligament(s) of knee, 190, 191
Comminution, as fracture pattern, 5
Compartment syndrome, 78, 86, 184, 212

Compound fracture(s), 8
Computerized (assisted) tomography, in diagnosis of trauma, 18
Condyle, lateral humeral, injury of, 74
Cortical bone, growth changes in, 2
Cruciate ligament(s), injury of, 198, 199
Cubitus valgus, 74
Cubitus varus, 68, 72, 78

Deformation, plastic, 5
Deformity(ies) angular, 99, 128, 162, 166
Dens, fracture of, 142, 143
Diaphysis, 3, 56, 66, 102–105, 118, 174, 175, 212, 213
Diastasis, of pubic symphysis, 152, 153
Disc, herniated, 150, 151
Dislocation(s), 24, 60, 184–187

Elbow injury(ies), classification of, 72–97
Embolism, fat, 9
Epicondyle, fracture of, 4, 80, 82
Epiphyseal fracture(s) classification of, 38
Epiphyseal ossification center, anatomy of, 4, 17
Epiphysiolysis, following fracture, 15, 40
Epiphysis, 4, 44, 45, 52, 54, 55, 58, 62, 74–83, 145, 182, 220–225

Facet joint(s), 144–149
Fat pad, 15
Fibula, distal, 216–225
Finger(s), dislocation of, 130, 131
Foot injury(ies), 226–241
Forearm fracture(s), 96–111

Genitourinary tract, injury of, 152
Greenstick fracture(s), 7, 64, 66
Growth arrest, 22, 24, 28, 34
Growth arrest (slowdown) lines, 16
Growth mechanism(s), 22–43

Hand injury(ies), 112–137
Head injury(ies), 11, 49
Heterotopic bone, 13
Hip dislocation, 160–163
Humerus, 60–83

Ilium, fracture of, 154–157
Immobilization, 9–11
Impaction, as fracture pattern, 2, 7, 68
Infection, 11, 36
Interphalangeal joint, of hand, 130, 131
Ischemia, following hip injury, 160–165
Ischium, fracture of, 158–159

Joint(s) dislocation of, 60, 86, 114, 122,
  130, 160, 184
Joint injury(ies), 30, 32

Knee, dislocation of, 184, 185
Knee injury(ies), 178–209

Lateral condyle, 74
Lateral epicondyle, 82, 83
Lateral malleolus, 224, 225
Leg length inequality, 10, 32, 34
Ligament(s), 190, 191, 198, 199

Magnetic resonance imaging, 21
Malleolus(i), fracture of, 5, 38, 224, 225
Mallet finger, 134, 135
Malrotation, 11
Malunion, 7, 11, 12, 30, 32
Meniscus, discoid, 196, 197
Metacarpals, fracture of, 118–121
Metacarpophalangeal dislocation, 122,
  123
Metaphysis, anatomy of, 4, 40
Metatarsal(s), injury of, 236, 237
Monteggia fracture-dislocation, 96, 97
Myelodysplasia, 46
Myositis ossificans, following trauma, 86

Nail, damage to, 136, 137
Navicula (carpal), fracture of, 112, 113
Neonate, injury in, 44, 60, 72
Nerve, peripheral injury in, 66, 68, 74, 82
Newborn, epiphyseal separation in, 44,
  72

Non-union, as fracture complication, 13,
  30, 42, 74

Obstetric fracture(s), 44, 60, 72
Odontoid process, 142, 143
Olecranon, 92, 93
Open injury(ies), 8, 42
Os trigonum, 228, 229
Osgood-Schlatter lesion, 38, 50
Ossification center, 22–43
Osteochondral fracture, 38, 39, 182, 183
Osteochondritis dissecans, 182
Osteogenesis imperfecta, 48
Osteomyelitis, 11, 36
Overgrowth, 10

Patella, bipartite, 192, 193
Pelvic injury(ies), 152–161
Periosteum, damage to, 1, 26, 42
Phalanx (phalanges), 122–137, 240, 241
Physeal injury(ies), 22–39
Physis, 4, 24, 34
Plastic deformation, 5, 6, 98, 99, 214,
  215
Pseudomonas, in foot puncture wounds,
  226, 227
Pulled elbow, 90, 91
Puncture wound, of foot, 226, 227

Radial head, anatomy of, 91
Radiology, adequate films in, 14
Radionuclide imaging, 18, 46
Radius, fracture of, 94, 95, 98–109
Ranvier, zone of, 36
Reduction, 9
Rotation, correction of, 7, 9

Scintigraphy, 18, 46, 51
Sleeve fracture, of patella, 194, 195
Slipped capital femoral epiphysis, 164,
  165
Spina bifida, 24, 46
Spine injury(ies), 44, 138–151
Spine, tibial, 198, 199
Sternoclavicular joint, 54, 55
Stress films, in diagnosis, 17, 31, 74
Stress fracture(s), 50, 84, 204, 214, 215
Synostosis, 42

Talus injury, 228, 229
Thumb, 114–117
Thurstan Holland sign, 26
Tibia injury, of diaphysis, 212–215
Tibial spine, 198, 199

Tibial tuberosity, 202–205
Tibial valgus, 40, 210, 211
Tibiofibular syndesmosis, 222
Tillaux fracture, 222, 223
Toddler's fracture, 214, 215
Torus fracture, 7, 64
Traction, 172, 174
Transverse lines of Park, 16
Triplane fracture, 220, 221
Trochanter, 168–171

Ulna fracture, 92–111
Urethra injury, 152

Vascular injury, 8, 19, 20, 68
Vasculature (vascularity), 40
Vertebra(e), 138–151
Volkmann's ischemia, 19

Wrist injury, 112, 113